Music, Science, and the R

Routledge Research in Music

Music, Science, and the Rhythmic Brain

Cultural and Clinical Implications

**Edited by Jonathan Berger
and Gabe Turow**

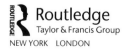
Routledge
Taylor & Francis Group

NEW YORK   LONDON

First published 2011
by Routledge
711 Third Avenue, New York, NY 10017

Simultaneously published in the UK
by Routledge
2 Park Square, Milton Park, Abingdon, Oxon OX14 4RN

*Routledge is an imprint of the Taylor & Francis Group,
an informa business*

First issued in paperback 2013

Typeset in Sabon by IBT Global.

Library of Congress Cataloging-in-Publication Data
    Music, science, and the rhythmic brain : cultural and clinical
implications / edited by Jonathan Berger and Gabe Turow.
        p. cm. — (Routledge research in music)
    Includes bibliographical references and index.
    1. Musical meter and rhythm—Physiological aspects.   2. Musical
meter and rhythm—Psychological aspects.   I. Berger, Jonathan,
1954–   II. Turow, Gabe, 1982–
    ML3820.M876 2011
    781'.11—dc22
    2011008070

ISBN13: 978-0-415-89059-5 (hbk)
ISBN13: 978-0-203-80529-9 (ebk)
ISBN13: 978-0-415-70948-4 (pbk)

Contents

PART I

Research on Rhythmic Entrainment in Music

PART II

Clinical Implications of Rhythmic Entrainment Research

Figures

Tables

Acknowledgments

This collection of essays is an outgrowth of the first two symposia on music and the brain which took place at Stanford University's Center for Computer Research in Music and Acoustics (CCRMA) in May 2006 and May 2007. These symposia marked the opening of the Center for Arts, Science and Technology (CAST) under the auspices of The Stanford Institute for Creativity and the Arts (SiCa).

Numerous people assisted in making both the symposia and this book possible. In addition to his technical and production skills, Michael Gubman contributed to the content and spirit of the symposia as well as provided editorial assistance and critical comments on many of the chapters in this volume. We are grateful for the enthusiastic support and encouragement of Moy Eng and Shireen Pasha from the Hewlett Foundation. We acknowledge the assistance of Sasha Leitman, Patricia Shroetter, and the entire CCRMA staff and community, and of Elisa Gomez Hird and the SiCa staff in producing the Symposia.

We thank Blair Bohanan for her careful proof-reading of this volume, Liz Seibert who faithfully reproduced numerous graphs and figures, and Elon Berger for formatting and editing assistance.

Editorial work on this volume was supported by a grant from the A. Jess Shensen Fund and by funding from the William and Flora Hewlett Foundation.

Those of us who were fortunate enough to know Tom Budzynski admired and greatly respected both his major pioneering work and his continuing technical and theoretical contributions in the fields of biofeedback and neurofeedback. The world is a little less bright now than it was before his departure on February 14th, 2011. He was a creative engineer, a scientist, a teacher, a clinician and a very likable man. It is characteristic of him that, near the end of his long and varied life, he was still continuing to make a contribution to knowledge in his field with the writing of his chapter in Music, Science, and the Rhythmic Brain.

Preface

This is a book about the effects of repetitive musical rhythm on the brain and nervous system. The topic integrates diverse fields, including ethnomusicology, psychology, neuroscience, anthropology, religious studies, music therapy, and human health. The volume, which originated in a symposium at Stanford University in 2007, discusses musical and biological rhythms, and in particular rhythmic entrainment, in a way that considers cultural context alongside theoretical research. The book also focuses on potential clinical and therapeutic implications of the laboratory research.

The book is divided into two parts. The first five chapters introduce aspects of rhythmic entrainment by researchers in ethnomusicology, cultural anthropology, and neuroscience. The chapters primarily review recent and historical lab experiments designed to tease out the mechanisms behind human entrainment to music. One of the central themes of this section concerns the effects of drumming and other rhythmic music on mental and bodily functioning. It is hypothesized that rhythmic music can have a dramatic impact on mental states, sometimes catalyzing profound changes in arousal, mood, and emotion. The experiments presented here make use of electroencephalography (EEG), galvanic skin response (GSR), and subjective measures to gain insight into how mental states are stimulated by rhythmic music, what their relationship is to the context of the experience, and demonstrate that these states are evoked in a consistent and reproducible fashion. A subset of these experiments was designed to investigate who among us seems to respond most strongly to music. These responders are termed 'deep listeners', and, it is proposed, may have unique physiologies that separate them from the rest of the music-enjoying population.

The later chapters in this section review some of the terminology crucial to the scientific study of rhythm, discuss EEG signal processing methods, and explore brainwave entrainment using modern statistical approaches. These techniques and concepts are vital to accurate and responsible experimentation and especially important given the complex phenomenology of many of the events being studied.

The second section of the book addresses select clinical applications of rhythmic entrainment. The section begins with a discussion of modern music therapy and the manner in which current work with rhythm and neu-roscience informs various interventions. The treatment of stroke, speech therapy, and movement therapy are emphasized. The next chapter explores binaural beat stimulation, a technology in which one tone is presented to one ear and a similar tone of slightly different frequency is presented to the other ear, creating an auditory beating effect for the listener that does not exist as a physical stimulus. This technique appears to be capable of systematically modifying ongoing brain activity, resulting in states of increased vigilance and altered mood. The following chapter illustrates the use of rhythmic music in combination with rhythmic light therapy, known as audio-visual stimulation (AVS). This multi-modal form of stimulation has been used to treat stroke, brain damage, dementia, and other cognitive impairments. This builds on the work presented in the early chapters of the book that suggest that rhythmic auditory stimulation can affect brain func-tioning and can systematically alter ongoing patterns of brainwave activ-ity. The final clinical chapter investigates the use of EEG driven AVS as an inexpensive, non-invasive, treatment for ADHD and learning disabilities in young people. Because the cognitive effects of this type of stimulation are similar to those of rhythmic music, its potential use in combination with music therapy is explored in some detail.

Part I

Research on Rhythmic Entrainment in Music

1 Introduction to Entrainment and Cognitive Ethnomusicology

Udo Will and Gabe Turow

ETHNOMUSICOLOGY AND COGNITIVE ETHNOMUSICOLOGY

Ever since their discovery in the early 20th century brain rhythms have fascinated the human mind and spurred a wide range of fascinating research aimed at understanding the functions of these rhythms at various levels. Brain rhythms are not only essential for organizing motor actions—for example in music-making—but also, as research in recent decades has indicated, for our cognition and for how we experience the world (for a good review on this: Buzsáki, 2006). Surprisingly, it seems that musicologists and ethnomusicologists, for whom, one might assume, rhythm would be a topic of foremost interest, have hardly taken note of this research, much less taken part in it.

For the most part this lack of interest can be attributed to the anti-scientific stance of the post-modern culturalism that came to dominate approaches in anthropology and ethnomusicology since the '60s. With the introduction and acceptance of the Schneider-Geertzian ideas about culture as an autonomous domain of arbitrary symbolic representations, action and social context lost their place in the research agenda—a radical transformation and departure from the model of their teacher, Parson's general theory of action. However, political and economic forces, social institutions, biological and physiological processes cannot be wished away, or simply assimilated into systems of knowledge and belief. Already one of Schneider's students, David Labby (1976:12), noted:

> The 'cultural analysis' that attempts to define the way people think but ignores the way people live . . . seems to me to be significantly misconceived . . . there is, properly speaking, no such thing as a distinct or separate 'cultural analysis'.

As we have argued elsewhere (Will, 2007), despite its magnitude and influence on contemporary cultural anthropology and ethnomusicology, this postmodernist approach is seriously biased and flawed by premises that are more rooted in modernist thinking than in alternatives to it—postmodernism as the elaborated logical continuation and extension of the modern, the cultural logic of the late capitalist condition. This is most evident in the objectification and materialization of the notion of culture, the resurgence of the notion of race, the acceptance of the illusory nature–culture divide, the ignorance of the human body, and the exclusive reliance on verbal accounts of actors' conscious thoughts. Indeed, in both the accounts of the cognitivists and the culturalists, biology (physiology) and culture are considered independent autonomous domains; this may be one of the central reasons why there has been little talk and exchange across the disciplines.

Though problems and limitations of the interpretive culturalist approach have been recognized early on even by postmodernist thinkers like V. Turner (Turner, 1987), this approach has been and still is dominant in ethnomusicology. Nevertheless, in recent years we see a variety of new topics and orientations emerging. As in other humanistic disciplines, such changes are in part motivated by the realization of the changing human life-world. Ethnomusicology not only has to take account of new types of music, new, technologies and conditions of music production and transmission, but is also facing changes in its working conditions in (see, e.g., the discussion on fieldwork in Wood, 2008) and for society. New roles and tasks for ethnomusicologists are sought, for example, within the emerging field of medical ethnomusicology, which aims to combine efforts of various experts, music and health specialists among them, to work on health and disease related issues in societies the world over (e.g., Barz, 2006). Guided by the collaboration of health sciences and healing arts, this field wants to engage knowledge from diverse research areas and domains of human life conventionally viewed as disparate, yet laden with potential benefits for an improved or vibrant quality of life, prevention of illness and disease, even cure and healing (from the liner notes, Koen, 2008).

In other recent developments in ethnomusicology, focus has been redirected towards music performances. There are indications of a shift from performance studies theory to practice (e.g., Keil, 1998) as well as a re-evaluation of the performative capabilities of ethnomusicologists (Bailey, 2008). There are also new developments towards more empirically oriented analyses of musical performances (see, e.g., various contributions in Stobart, 2008). These latter developments are emerging in response to reflections on the current state of ethnomusicology and its relationship to other disciplines, in particular, the sciences. Quite a few scholars have realized that the culturalist position has not only led to theoretical problems and practical impasses in their own discipline (Will, 2007) but also to an unfortunate insulation from developments in other disciplines that are of utmost relevance for overcoming those difficulties and for reconnecting cultural studies with relevant discourses in other disciplines.

Developments in cognitive sciences since the '80s suggest that we are witnessing a breakdown of concepts at the very basis of the culturalists' approach. They show that human cognition is not independent of the body (e.g., works of Johnson, Kay & McDaniel, Barsalou, Damasio), that meaning is grounded in the interactions of organisms with and within their environment, not in arbitrary socio-cultural conventions (e.g., works of Varela, Johnson, Rizzolatti, Ramachandran), and that the working of the brain is largely shaped by experience (works of Freeman, Merzenich, Varela). These developments make clear that the old dichotomies between nature and nurture, biology and culture, the individual and universal have lost their explanatory significance and can no longer be maintained. For both the cultural and natural sciences these developments pose serious challenges as cognitivists and culturalists are losing their foundational concepts. Furthermore, they call not only for extensive conceptual and methodological changes in both fields, but also for close cooperation and cross-disciplinary exchange.

Cooperation is especially needed in the domain of music that, since the mid '90s, was discovered by the cognitive sciences as a new area of research, complementary to language studies. This has led to the publication of a number of special volumes dedicated to the cognitive processing of music by the New York Academy of Sciences, by Nature Neuroscience, and reviews, editorials, and essays in major scientific journals.

However, this surge of cognitive studies on music comes with a concern. *The research seems to be fundamentally biased towards Western music*: Though lip service is frequently paid to the importance of variety in music cultures, experimental and clinical studies almost exclusively utilize subjects from Western cultures and music based on the Western classical tradition. Clearly, as Ian Cross (2003) has put it, the foundational categories of theorized Western musical practices form the basis for most perceptual and cognitive theory and experimentation about music. This is of concern because Western Classical music has developed in close connection with a specific writing system and many of its principles are different from those of non-Western musics (for details and examples: Blacking, 1961; Arom, 1997; Will, 1999; Cross, 2003). To arrive at a generalizable understanding of cognitive processing of music, cross-cultural studies are needed and this is where the experience of ethnomusicology is a condition sine qua non. This experience, however, cannot just be borrowed. *Extensive interdisciplinary cooperation is needed for an integration of cognitive and ethnographic research programs.* If, in terms of the revised conceptualizations mentioned above, understanding situated music making requires more than analysis of verbal accounts, then we need to consider additional explanatory variables, like for example, spatial and temporal structures of musicians actions, their physiological states of mind and body, etc. The significant methodological problem ethnomusicology has to address is: how to study these variables in an ecologically valid manner. This is what we would consider the proper domain of cognitive ethnomusicology, and the case of *musical entrainment* is an example par excellence of the active, contributing role ethnomusicology can and would have to play in order to make this approach work.

Entrainment is a concept coming from complex systems theory that posits that two or more independent, autonomous oscillatory processes, if and when they can interact, influence (entrain) each other mutually, and the degree of influence is dependent on the coupling force(s). Complex systems theory, however, is ignorant as to what constitutes a coupling factor. It is here where the expertise of the discipline applying the concept—ethnomusicology in our example—is needed in order to identify the coupling factors at work in specific musical contexts. Entrainment is a concept with a considerable history—first identified by the Dutch physicist Christiaan Huygens in 1665 and subsequently applied widely in mathematics and the physical, biological, and social sciences. It is a process that manifests in many ways, some of which involve human agency or cognition.

This principle posits that any two oscillators will entrain if allowed to interact for long enough. Huygens discovered this phenomenon during an experiment with pendulum clocks: He set them each in motion and found that when he returned the next day, the sway of their pendulums had all synchronized. He extrapolated that entrainment is a ubiquitous natural phenomenon that manifests via the conservation of energy during the interaction of closely related rhythmic cycles. *The tendency for rhythmic processes or oscillations to adjust in order to match other rhythms has been described in a wide variety of systems and over a wide range of time scales (i.e., periodicities):* from fireflies illuminating in synchrony, through human individuals adjusting their speech rhythms to match each other in conversation, to the movement of electric driers placed in close proximity, to the way that a room of clapping people will spontaneously fall into rhythm (Neda, Ravasz, Brechet, Vicsek, & Barabsi, 2000). Examples have been claimed from the relatively fast frequency oscillations of brainwaves to periods extending over months and years, and in organisms from the simplest to the most complex as well as in the behavior of inorganic materials and systems.

Strangely, entrainment has had relatively little impact to date on studies of music, where it might be thought particularly relevant. We believe that this concept could have a particularly significant impact if applied to musicological and ethnomusicological research because it offers a new approach to understanding music making and music perception as an integrated, embodied, and interactive process, and can therefore shed light on many issues central to musicological thought. Entrainment will be of special relevance to research orientations for which performance of and listening to music are the focus of interest, as well as for those interested in understanding the impact of musical rhythms and rhythmic stimulation on the human body and mind.

SENSORY STIMULATION AS RITUAL TECHNOLOGY

From Tibetan Buddhist rites to Middle Eastern Sufi rituals, from Siberian, European, and South American Shamanic traditions to Caribbean Hatian ceremonies, and in Jewish and Christian worship in America and elsewhere, repetitive musical rhythm is a common feature in religious practice (Eliade, 1964; Keil & Feld, 1994). The ubiquity of this form of stimulation in religious contexts suggests that it is more than ornamental or simply traditional.

Mantra recitation, perhaps the most common rhythmic prayer, has been scientifically investigated in some detail. A mantra is any string of words that are repeated over and over again with the intention of inducing a meditative state or of inspiring religious experience. Reciting a mantra can be an intense and consistent form of rhythmic auditory stimulation. Mantra recitation has been shown to reduce anxiety levels and increase alpha power (Lee et al., 1997), induce relaxation (Janowiak & Hackman, 1994), lower blood pressure (Seer & Raeburn, 1980), and induce an increase in theta and delta waves (Stigsby, Rodenberg, & Moth, 1981).

Rhythmic prayer also has interesting effects. In a study comparing recitation of the Ave Maria prayer to the yogic mantra Om Mani Padme Hum, scientists observed that both types of rhythmic recitation equally slowed respiration and caused striking, powerful, and synchronous increases in existing cardiovascular rhythms (Bernardi et al., 2001).

Tibetan Buddhists have a long and well-documented history of using musical instruments like drums and bells to help enter, deepen, and sustain meditation during rituals. Jonathan Goldman, a lecturer for the International Society for Music and Medicine who has studied with the Dalai Lamas Chanting Gyuto and Gyume Monks, explains that:

> Tibetan bells, or Ting-Sha's, have been utilized in Buddhist meditation practice for many centuries. An examination reveals that the two bells, which are rung together, are slightly out of tune with each other. Depending upon the bells, the difference tones between them create ELFs (extremely low frequency oscillations in the theta and delta range) somewhere between 4 and 8 cycles per second. This falls within the range of the brainwaves created during meditation or sleep, and [may] help shift the brain to these frequencies. (Goldman, 2004)

The ELFs Goldman describes produce a modulation that continues until the sound of one of the bells decays.

Tibetan singing bowls produce a similar effect. Dragging a wooden stick around the rim of a singing bowl creates a sustained complex tone characterized by an ethereal ringing with audible frequency modulation, resulting from rotating quadropoles created by the interaction of the puja (stick) and the bowl (Octavia, Luis, & Antunes, 2005). This pulsing remains at a constant tempo as long as the bowl is vibrating at an even rate. In addition to the friction of the rubbed puja, beating can also be produced from the bowl by striking it on its side and allowing it to ring. These bowls are used as an adjunct to quiet meditation, and monks will often chant along with the ELFs.[1]

The damaru, another common Tibetan prayer instrument, is a two-headed hand-held drum. It has two beads attached to two strings connected to the opposite sides of the body of the drum. When it is rotated between the palms, it is easy to produce an even beat at a similar tempo to the pulsations of a singing bowl. These drums are used in many Tibetan meditative settings to supply a consistent beat for prayer. There are hundreds of examples of such instruments used in similar ways around the world.

ETHNOMUSICOLOGICAL DEBATE
ON MOOD-ALTERING MUSIC

Among anthropologists and ethnomusicologists, there has been debate since the early 1950s about the extent to which different psychological and social-environmental factors play into the induction of trance states in a variety of ritual contexts. Though this seems like an unusual subject of inquiry, trance states are fascinating examples of altered states of attention, arousal, and mood. Specifically, the question: *Can music (alone or in context) induce trance?* has had a wide variety of answers from different researchers. This provides an interesting inroad to the dialogue on music's many observed effects on the nervous system.

Gilbert Rouget has made the most intense effort of any anthropologist in the last quarter century to explore the issues surrounding trance-inducing music, summarized in his book *Music and Trance: A Theory of Relations between Music and Possession*, originally published in 1980 (English publication in 1985). Following the first third of the book, which explores many ritual trances involving music, Rouget reviews the anthropological literature on the neurophysiological effects of drumming and other repetitive auditory stimulation.

The centerpiece of his discussion is Andrew Neher's laboratory study of auditory driving (Neher, 1961). *Auditory driving refers to the hypothesized ability of repetitive rhythmic auditory stimuli to alter brainwave activity in a one-to-one relationship.* For example, if a subject hears drum rhythms at 8 beats per second, it is hypothesized that one's brainwaves will be influenced by this stimulus, producing more activity at 8Hz and possibly influencing other brainwave frequency bands, thereby altering brain activity as a whole. Neher's study and this hypothesis were the basis for much of the speculation concerning the biological mechanisms of trance in the years between 1962 and 1980.

Rouget (1985) surveys Neher's influence on the ethnomusicological dialogue starting in 1955 with Dr. Charles Pidoux, a physician and ethnopsychiatrist who studied possession cults in Mali. Pidoux hypothesized that drumbeats might act upon "different levels of the neural axis."[2] In 1961 Neher published his laboratory data on auditory driving, followed in 1962 with an article on the ramifications of his finding for the field of anthropology. In 1967, Rodney Needham published an article in Man entitled "Percussion and Transition," where he seems to build on Neher's recent papers. Needham asserts "All over the world . . . percussion . . . permits or accompanies communication with the other world." The problem then, according to Needham, was to discover the exact relationship between the concept of spiritual existence (i.e., non-ordinary states of consciousness) and this "non-cultural affective appeal of percussion."[3]

Needham seemed to view percussion, regardless of rhythm, melody, or repetition, as the key to the induction of trance. Convinced that *the sound* was key, he continues, "There is no doubt that sound-waves have neural and organic effects on human beings, irrespective of the cultural formation of the latter" and adds that trance occurs as a result of disturbances brought about by the sounds of the drums "in the inner ear, an organ which modulates postural attitudes, muscular tonus, breathing rhythms, heartbeat, blood pressure, feelings of nausea, and certain eye reflexes."[4]

In 1968 W.C. Sturtevant wrote in a letter to the editor of Man headed "Categories, Percussion and Physiology," that the effects of trance and music are so widespread because some universal psychological or physiological mechanism is at work.[5] Similarly, Anthony Jackson took on a brain-phenomena line of reasoning in his article "Sound and Ritual" (1968) when he wrote that "since the brain is a common denominator to all mankind, it follows that what is true at the neuro-physiological level must be universally true."[6] In 1972, Sheila S. Walker writes in "Ceremonial Spirit Possession in Africa and Afro-America:"

> the most fundamental element of possession is the presence of neurophysiological changes, [and these] are most frequently produced by sensory bombardment, usually in the form of sonic driving [reference to Neher, 1962] of the drum rhythms.[7]

She adds later,

> the hypnotic state [trance] is triggered by the altered state of consciousness and changes in body ego produced by the neurophysiological effects of the rhythmic drumming.[8]

Additionally, Rouget notes that Neher's theory has found a certain reputation as indicated by the

> pages Raymond Prince (1968, 133–135) devoted to it in his article on encephalography and research into possession states, by the allusions

made to it during the 1968 Paris Colloquium by various ethnologists, and by the reference T. F. Johnston (1972, 30) makes to it in his article on possession music among the Tsonga, in which it is clear that he, too, regards it as a given.[9]

But in the subsequent discussion, Rouget raises a series of objections against Neher's theory and its interpretation by the above authors. Some of his objections are obviously unqualified and inappropriate, for instance when he simply dismisses Neher's 'appareil scientifique'—a reference to Neher's 1961 paper—as 'pseudo-scientific', or when he questions the Fisher's exact probability test in a dire pun that only shows that Rouget is not well versed in statistical reasoning.

Other points are, however, absolutely crucial and reach beyond Rouget's specific critique of Neher's 1962 paper. They are certainly worth consideration whenever laboratory findings concerning physiological reactions to music are used to (re-)interpret ethnographical research. Rouget's main points are:

1. Lab experiments show certain physiological reactions, but the link between these reactions and the states of trance as described by ethnologists remains obscure especially if subjects did not fall into trance during the lab experiments.
2. To construct an analogy between auditory driving results and reports from photic driving experiments, where altered and/or epileptic states have been reported, is unconvincing on the basis of the known differences between the two sensory systems as well as the data Neher reports.
3. Ethnographic reports indicate that drum rhythms are not a sufficient criterion to evoke trance: Many ceremonies that use drum rhythms do not produce trance states.
4. Ethnographic evidence indicates that drum rhythms are also not a necessary element to produce trance states.

In the years since the publication of Rouget's *La Musique et la Transe*, even with the development of many new technologies to investigate the real-time functioning of the human brain, vaguely defined physiological theories have largely remained dominant in the ethnomusicological discourse on music's influences on the brain and nervous system, and no significant challenges to the auditory driving hypothesis have arisen. It is possible that the lack of subsequent progress to either debunk Neher's theory or propose a detailed alternative may have been due to a lack of interdisciplinary efforts, interest in the questions themselves, or research funding to investigate these types of phenomena. However, with the current robust and growing interest in neuroscientific studies on music we see promising changes, and a recent cross-disciplinary study that replicated Neher's experimental paradigm

(Will & Berg, 2007)[10] has produced some new insights that may contribute to an improved understanding of these issues.

Moreover, in the last decade many ethnographic observations on the effects of drumming on the brain and nervous system have gained increasing support from other disciplines. There is a new and growing body of research suggesting that drumming can affect a wide range of physical conditions, mental illnesses, and personality disorders (Friedman, 2001). Rhythmic auditory stimulation has been demonstrated to improve immune function (Bittman et al., 2001; Wachiuli et al., 2007), enhance hypnotic susceptibility (Maurer, Kumar, Woodside, & Pekala, 1997; Szabó, 2004), increase relaxation, improve mood, and help manage stress (Bittman, Bruhn, Stevens, Westengard, & Umbach, 2003; Bittman et al., 2004), and induce altered states of consciousness (Mandell, 1980). In addition, many of the modern physiological and subjective reports on the effects of sustained rhythmic drumming parallel and intersect with research describing the dynamics of altered states of consciousness (Winkelman, 1997, 2000), states of meditation (Walton & Levitsky, 1994), and hypnosis (Maurer et al., 1997; Szabó, 2004; Woodside et al., 1997; Winkelman, 2003).

Today, some areas of ethnomusicology are moving from a humanistic phenomenological discipline towards a scientific framework that can incorporate facets of neuroscience and cognitive psychology in order to better answer questions that are of key importance. There is still no clear answer as to why drumming, among other rhythmic stimuli, seems to be able to induce dramatic affective and arousal changes in so many different kinds of people. Within this context, the concept of entrainment can act as a fascinating lens. The rest of this introductory chapter will be devoted to the scholarly dialogue on entrainment and its relevance to understanding the many effects of musical rhythm on human beings.

ENTRAINMENT IN DETAIL

As explained above, *entrainment describes an action whereby two oscillatory processes interact with each other in such a way that they adjust towards and eventually lock into a common phase and/or periodicity.* Specifically, there are two basic components involved in all instances of entrainment:

1. *There are always two or more autonomous rhythmic processes or oscillators involved.* "Autonomous" means that if the two oscillators are separated, that is, if they do not interact, they must still be able to oscillate: The oscillations must be active processes requiring an internal source of energy. In other words, none of the oscillations (or the rhythmic processes) should be caused through the interaction. Resonance, for example, is not to be considered entrainment: If a

tuning fork producing sound waves in a resonance box is removed, the oscillations in the box also cease. That is an important point, because it alerts us to the possibility that the mere observation of synchronized behavior or synchronous variation in two variables does not necessarily imply entrainment. This is also the reason why we prefer the term entrainment over synchronization, although the latter has been considerably promoted in the last decade through well known publications like Steven Strogatz's *Sync, the emerging science of spontaneous order* (2003) or Pikovsky, Rosenblum, & Kurths' *Synchronization. A universal concept in nonlinear science* (2001).

2. *The oscillators must interact.* There are a variety of different forms of possible interactions or coupling, but in the majority of cases this interaction is weak, as demonstrated by Huygen's pendulum clock example. Strong coupling, on the other hand, puts too strong a limitation on the oscillators, and they lose their 'individuality' (for example, if one were to make circular movements with both arms, consider how these movements would be limited if both hands held on to the same stick). *The interactions between oscillators can be unidirectional* as, for example, in the case of human entrainment to diurnal cycles. Here the entraining oscillator (diurnal cycle) is not affected by the entrained oscillator (human being). However, in most cases of entrainment between living beings we are dealing with bi-directional or multi-directional interactions. As will become clear from the following discussion, identification and quantified description of the weak interactions is one of the biggest challenges in entrainment research.

The wide range of entrainment phenomena is not based on a single physical process. Rather, *the concept of entrainment describes a shared tendency of a wide range of physical and biological systems: namely, the coordination of temporally structured events through interaction.* In principle, it is easy to see how entrainment is relevant to music. If a musicologist were asked to suggest a familiar example of a temporally structured event, it is likely that music, or some social or ritual event mediated through music, would quickly come to mind. Examples of rhythmic coordination to and through music, such as a foot tapping to the beat of a song, are equally easy to think of. However, so far entrainment studies in musicology are limited to a few examples, and it may be beneficial for musical applications to take into account the wider context of entrainment in human biological and social functioning.

Examples of endogenous or naturally occurring rhythms within the human body include the heart beat, blood circulation, respiration, locomotion, eyes blinking, secretion of hormones, and female menstrual cycles, among others. It has been suggested that all human movements are inherently rhythmic. Jones writes that "All human performance can be evaluated within a rhythmic framework,"[11] whereas Bernieri, Reznick, and Rosenthal suggest that, "human behavior is understood to occur rhythmically and therefore can be described in terms of cycles, periods, frequencies, and amplitudes."[12]

As we will see, these endogenous rhythmic processes may interact in many different ways within an individual or interpersonally. These two types of entrainment, self-entrainment and interpersonal entrainment, engage different sets of coupling factors. In particular, entrainment to and through music needs to be seen as a particular case of entrainment in social interaction, and its specific qualities need to be identified and explored.

METER, TIMING AND ATTENTION

In music research, we have already seen an entrainment perspective adopted in the study of musical meter, particularly in the 1990s. Instead of looking for musical cues transmitted from performer to listener as the sole determinants of time and meter percepts, music psychologists have begun to apply an entrainment model in which rhythmic processes endogenous to the listener entrain to cues in the musical sound (Large & Kolen, 1994). Although there is much to explore in this area, the entrainment model seems to reflect the cognitive processes much better than previous models of metrical perception. Some recent work also points to new perspectives offered by the entrainment concept in the study of proto-musical behavior in infants, and in the evolution of musical behavior in the human species (Trevarthen, 1999; Merker, 2000).

More generally, several cognitive psychologists hold that perception, attention, and expectation are all rhythmic processes subject to entrainment (Large & Jones, 1999; see also Ward, 2002, 2003). In other words, even when a person is only listening to speech or music, their perceptions and expectations will be coordinated by their entrainment to what they hear. Entrainment is fundamental then, not just to coordinate with others, but even to perceive, react to, and enjoy music. Music, as an external oscillator entraining our internal oscillators, has the potential to affect not only our sense of time but also our sense of being in the world. Moreover, it is clear that people exercise a significant measure of self-control in negotiating musical entrainment. These ideas are essentially informed by the work of Mari Riess Jones and her co-workers, as published since 1976. Some basic assumptions about entrainment that we have already presented above are quite similarly expressed in these studies. Jones assumes that human beings are inherently rhythmical, with tunable perceptual rhythms that can entrain to stimulus (or event) patterns in the physical world. In other words, she postulates a propensity for an individual's endogenous rhythms to synchronize with perceived and expected rhythmic processes (Jones, 1976; Jones & Boltz, 1989).

Another basic premise of Jones' theory is the assumption that many of the time structures perceived in real-world events are patterned in coherent and hierarchical ways (Jones, 1976). According to Jones, a hierarchical time structure is one in which

> the temporal distribution of markers [event onsets and relative stress] reveals nested time levels that are consistently related to one another by ratio or additive time transformations.[13]

Examples of additive time transformations include gradual changes in velocity, such as musical tempo changes, or changes occurring with a shift in physical momentum, as when a person breaks into a run from a casual walk. Most musical meters are examples of simple ratio relations between at least two distinct but nested time levels: "One is a referent time level, the beat period, and the other is a higher order period based on a fixed number of beat periods, the measure."[14]

Nested time levels in music may extend upward from the smallest subdivisions of a beat, to a beat level, to a measure, to a phrase, to a period, to large order forms. Percussion instructors often teach players to focus on the beat with the beat, referring to the simplest rhythm that lies at the center of any complex pattern.[15] By reducing the pattern to its simplest components in each rhythmic cycle, the player's attention can be anchored, even when executing highly complex musical phrases. Shifting attention between these cyclical layers of timing is one of the central and most difficult tasks for any musician.

One important aspect of entrainment theory is that, in many regards, it is a unifying concept, a concept with the potential to cut across disciplinary boundaries and to form a coherent basis applicable in various disciplines. It permits linkages between the cultural and the biological as well as the individual and the social, and it offers a new approach to understanding human action and perception as an integrated, embodied, and interactive process. In many disciplines, the perceived separation and opposition between nature and culture has slowly been recognized as an unfortunate and misleading byproduct of Western metaphysics that has dominated anthropological theorizing since the end of the 19th century (Jackson, 1989; Strathern, 1992; Becker, 2001; Will, 2007).

However, the development of alternative approaches has been slow and hesitant. An initial attempt towards overcoming the culture/nature divide in anthropology was the reintroduction in the 1970s of the body, the recognition that the human body is not able to be dissociated from the mind nor is the human mind a disembodied creative force (e.g., V. Turner, J. Blacking). During this period, research in brain sciences was largely dominated by a 'cognitivistic'—computational orientation (predicated on an analogy between the workings of the human brain and computer processing). This direction has been and still is criticized for neglecting or omitting the affective–emotional and bodily existence of humans, as well as eliminating contextual elements—a direction not well equipped to overcome the nature/culture dichotomy.

COUPLING FACTORS

During the last few decades, however, cognitive science saw the emergence of new and powerful paradigms—connectionism, autopoiesis, enaction/embodiment—as well as new orientations like neuro-phenomenology, that offer promising alternatives to the standard cognitivistic approach. In these approaches, cognition is understood as embodied action: bodily actions under brain control modify the brain through sensation, perception and learning, thereby incorporating the world through experience, not through information in the form of external symbols and internal representations. For a living being, the meaning of this or that interaction is not prescribed from the outside or arbitrarily set (from the inside), it is the result of the organization and the history of the living system itself. Furthermore, the enactive approach is based on situated, embodied agents and essentially comprises the ongoing coupling of the agent with its environment, fundamentally mediated by sensorimotor activities. It is this core notion of structural coupling (Varela, 1988; Varela, Thompson, & Rosch, 1991) that, from the perspective of the new neurosciences, dissolves the old nature/culture divide by showing that neither human biology nor human environment (culture, society) can be understood without the other. Moreover, for any approach in which structural coupling is a central element, interaction with the environment necessarily includes a supra-individual dimension. As for humans, the interaction with the environment is most importantly an interaction with conspecies: This dimension is essentially a social one. From this perspective, it can then be considered that the human brain has evolved as an organ of social organization (Freeman, 1995; Nunez, 1997).[16]

The concept of structural coupling links directly with entrainment theory where coupling strength (between oscillatory processes) is a crucial factor determining entrainment effects, and refers to the kind and degree of interactions with the human and non-human environment that influence entrainment. But the factors that affect coupling strength are not predefined by entrainment theory and have to be identified by the applying disciplines (e.g., ethnomusicology). Apart from biological factors like age (McAuley, Jones, Holub, Johnston, & Miller, 2006), psychological and cultural factors can also act as regulators of coupling strength. For example, our bodily responses to music are influenced by familiarity with the music as well as by musical training, cultural practices, and even belief systems. For example, in our entrainment research on Indian alap (Widdess, Will, & Clayton, 2005)—a section in Indian raga performances that, according to theory, is performed without a fixed pulse—some participants claimed not to be able to tap to examples of alap because it is not supposed to have a pulse, though most participants had no difficulties tapping along with this music. Cultural factors have been shown to influence entrainment within individual performers, such as cases where one individual performs multiple rhythmic actions, as in the instance of a singer who accompanies her/himself on an instrument (Clayton, Sager, & Will, 2005). Entrainment research is also elucidating how socio-communicative factors influence entrainment between individuals, establishing the link between the individual and the social by integrating human interaction.

RHYTHM AND AFFECTIVE STATES

Entrainment likely has considerable implications for another link that bridges the biological and the cultural, the link between rhythms and emotional, affective states, although this path has not yet been explored in depth. One of the problems facing this direction of research is that rhythm and emotions are rarely conceptualized in a commensurable way. On the other hand, abundant theoretical and practical links between music and affective states are evidenced by various music cultures around the globe. In addition, the efficacy of music therapy for the treatment of emotional disorders such as anxiety and depression has been demonstrated in a growing body of clinical research.[17] Yet, very little, if any, theory is available to account for this efficacy. (There are some developing scientific accounts of the music-therapeutic use of rhythm, like that of M. Thaut and colleagues, but they relate primarily to sensorimotor processes and generally leave out the question of affect and emotion).[18]

BRAINWAVE SYNCHRONIZATION AND ENTRAINMENT

The term entrainment, in the specific sense of frequency-following, is also widely used in connection with brainwaves. The technique of recording electrical activity of the human brain from the scalp originated in 1875 with Richard Caton's observations and was developed into electroencephalography by Hans Berger in the late 1920s. Berger found that the recorded activity can be described in terms of four frequency bands: delta (1–4Hz), theta (4–8Hz), alpha (8–12Hz), and beta (12–30Hz) waves. The electrical activity that is recorded in electroencephalograms (EEGs) is largely attributable to postsynaptic potentials (PSPs; i.e., graded potentials produced by synaptic activities, that eventually lead to firing of neurons) in cell bodies and dendrites of cortical neurons (Lopes da Silva & Storm van Leeuwen, 1978).

Neurons of the human brain, the gray matter, come in two principal arrangements: Layered, they form a cortex, and in non-layered agglomerations they form a nucleus. Two cortices, the cerebral and cerebellar cortex, form the surface layer of the human brain; nuclei are located beneath the cortex and in the brain stem. The columnar arrangement of neurons in the cerebral cortex facilitates summation of these potentials and their registration at the scalp. However, other geometric arrangements of neuronal assemblies can lead to extracellular attenuation or even cancellation. Therefore, not all activities of brain cells can be recorded in the EEG. The regular spontaneous EEG components are thought to be due to post-synaptic potentials (PSPs) synchronized by discharges from deep nuclei (e.g., thalamus) and the degree of synchronicity is reflected in the amplitude and form of the EEG (Lopes da Silva, 1991). If cortical activity is synchronous over a larger area it produces larger potentials (e.g., Cooper, Winter, Crow, & Walter, 1965). On the other hand, desynchronization of the EEG and reduction of its amplitudes presumably reflects increased interaction of several neuronal sub-populations engaging in cooperative activities.

Despite persisting uncertainties about the actual neuronal mechanisms that generate EEG (i.e., electroencephalogram) waves, and notwithstanding the fact that EEGs are incomplete records of neuronal activities in the brain, it has been obvious since Berger's days that EEGs reflect certain mental states. A dominance of low-amplitude beta waves (14–30Hz) is observed in busy and alert states, whereas alpha waves (8–12Hz) with larger amplitudes dominate in a relaxed, inattentive state (Berger, 1929).

In the early days of EEG research, it was also discovered that some of the alpha and beta waves could be synchronized to the frequency of an external, bright strobe light stimulus. The English neurosurgeon Gray Walter was the first to report that at certain specific frequencies of the external stimulus, his subjects would enter trance-like states where they began to experience deep peacefulness, dream-like visions, and other unexpected sensations (Walter, 1953). Later it was discovered that not only strobe lights but also rhythmic noises could produce such effects. Although these phenomena are far from being fully understood, they do indicate that external stimuli are able to affect brain states.

A first theoretical explanation of alpha waves on the basis of an entrainment model was attempted in the early '50s by Norbert Wiener. At that time little was known about the nature of oscillatory activity in the brain, and Wiener thought that the dominant frequency band, the alpha waves, was an essential clock mechanism for coordinating neural activity in perceptual and cognitive processing. His main idea was that a precise and reliable reference clock could be created through the interactions of a large set of sloppy clock oscillators that would lead to spontaneous synchronization across the set. His model predicted that if entrainment were producing the alpha peak in the EEG, then it should show a distribution with central peaks and marked dips on both sides of the peak—the dips being produced by attraction or pulling of neighboring frequencies towards the main peak frequency. Wiener published these ideas in a 1958 monograph entitled *Nonlinear problems in random theory*, but he did not succeed in developing a working mathematical model before his death in 1964. Current understanding of alpha waves no longer supports the view that they are generated through frequency-pulling from adjacent frequency bands (e.g., Başar, Başar-Eroglu, Karakas, & Schürmann, 2000).

There is ample evidence that the phenomenon of synchronization forms an important working mechanism of the brain and can be understood as a reflection of the cooperative activity of neurons within distributed assemblies.[19] This phenomenon entails two fundamental ideas:

- At least certain types of neural assemblies are characterized by the synchronous activity of their constituent neurons.
- The different EEG frequency components reveal synchronies relating to different perceptual, motor or cognitive states (Anokhin, Lutzenberger, & Birbaumer, 1999; Başar, Başar-Eroglu, Karakas, & Schürmann, 2000; Burgess & Gruzelier, 1997; Eckhorn et al., 1988; Engel, Konig, Kreiter, & Singer, 1991; Klimesch, 1999; Klimesch, Schimke, & Schwaiger, 1994; Miltner, Braun, Arnold, Witte, & Taub, 1999; Rodriguez et al., 1999; Tallon-Baudry, Bertrand, & Fischer, 2001; Tallon, Bertrand, Bouchet, & Pernier, 1995).

These two concepts find abundant support in recent studies of animal and human neurophysiology, for example those demonstrating increased power in the beta and gamma bands of EEG signals (i.e., frequencies above 13Hz) during perceptual or visuomotor tasks (Aoki, Fetz, Shupe, Lettich, & Ojemann, 1996; Keil, Muller, Ray, Gruber, & Elbert, 1999; Muller et al., 1996).

The degree of frequency-specific synchronization or coherence is also seen as an indicator of more general brain states. It has been found that the degree of coherence is lower in Alzheimer's patients, comatose subjects, and in brain-injured subjects, whereas it is higher in mentally retarded persons, during sleep, and during epileptic seizures. In between these extremes, intermediate levels of coherence for normal functioning have been described (Silberstein, 1995).

SENSORY STIMULATION AND SYNCHRONIZATION TO THE ENVIRONMENT

A central focus of this volume is on a subgroup of synchronization phenomena, those that occur in response to external rhythmic stimuli. The human body and brain are extremely sensitive to rhythmic activity in the environment, and can become synchronized to it on many levels, even when entrainment, in the sense of mutually impacting and interacting oscillators, is not necessarily ongoing. Sleep-wake cycles synchronize to the 24-hour phases of light and dark, and women's menstrual cycles synchronize when they live in groups. Respiration (Haas, Distenfeld, & Axen, 1986), motor movements (Safranek, Koshland, & Raymond, 1982; Thaut, Schleiffers, & Davis, 1992; Thaut, McIntosh, Prassas, & Rice, 1992, 1993; McIntosh, Thaut, & Rice, 1996), and the subtle body movements of people in conversation will synchronize (Condon, 1975) to rhythmic auditory stimuli. Brainwave synchronization to repetitive tactile stimuli occurs in cats (Pompeiano, 1962), monkeys (Walter & Adey, 1966), and humans (Namerow, 1974), and to low-level, low-frequency electrical and VHF fields in cats and monkeys (Gavalas, Walter, Hamer, & Adey, 1970). Moreover, for a long time it has been known that flashing lights can evoke EEG rhythms related to the stimulus frequency (Adrian & Matthews, 1934). In early EEG research it was also observed that flashing light stimuli at certain frequencies may even induce seizures in susceptible individuals (Walter, Dovey, & Shipton, 1946). These EEG responses to flashing light, also known as the photic driving response (PDR) or steady state visual evoked potential, is frequently used in routine clinical EEG examinations, and for investigating neurological disorders (Takahashi, 1987; Coull & Pedley, 1978; Duffy, Iyer, & Surwillo, 1989).

Since the discovery of the PDR, it has also been suggested that audio stimuli and combined audio-visual stimuli might have comparable clinical importance. Whereas pure audio stimulation received little attention in the 1950s and '60s, many subsequent studies focused on the ability of combined audio-visual stimulation (AVS) to induce relaxation and hypnosis (reviewed in Morse, 1993). Others have reported AVS to be effective for relieving a diversity of pain symptoms (Solomon, 1985), treating dental anxiety (Morse, 1993), premenstrual syndrome (Noton, 1997), fibromyalgia (Mueller, Donaldson, Nelson, & Layman, 2001) and for alleviating the cognitive dysfunctions associated with closed-head injury (Montgomery, Ashley, Burns, & Russell, 1994) and strokes (Russell, 1997; Rozelle & Budzynski, 1995; also see Chapter 10). Micheletti (1999) found AVS effective in improving cognitive and behavioral measures in children with attention deficit hyperactivity disorder (ADHD). Carter and Russell (1993) reported significant improvement in cognitive and behavioral functioning through repeated AVS sessions in learning disabled boys[20], and comparable results have been reported by Joyce and Siever (2000). It has also been suggested that an increase in EEG synchrony through biofeedback training could be used to normalize the synchronization deviations seen in dyslexic and head injured subjects (Hoffman, Stockdale, Hicks, & Schwaninger, 1995; Evans & Park, 1996).

The photic driving response is most reliable with a stimulus rate corresponding to the subject's peak alpha frequency (Toman, 1941; Townsend, Lubin, & Naitoh, 1975). Recent studies have shown, however, that AVS activates a diverse range of EEG frequencies beyond the primary sensory cortices and outside of the frequency of stimulation. Using low-frequency theta AVS, Dieter and Weinstein (1995) described a significant increase of delta and theta activity in frontal, central, and parietal regions. In a study of 13 college students, Timmermann, Lubar, Rasey, & Frederick (1999) found that effects of AVS were widely distributed across the scalp, and that AVS at a subject's dominant alpha frequency had no effect in the alpha band, but significantly increased power in the delta, theta, and beta bands. Stimulation at twice the dominant alpha frequency significantly increased theta, alpha, and beta power. Differences in coherence following photic driving have been described between normal subjects and patients with Alzheimer's disease (Wada et al., 1998), schizophrenia (Wada, Nanbu, Kikuchi, Koshino, & Hashimoto, 1998), and between genders (Wada, Nanbu, Kadoshima, & Jiang, 1996). Effects of auditory, visual, and combined auditory-visual stimulation on coherence in normal subjects are reported by Frederick and colleagues (1999).

AUDITORY DRIVING

Considerable research has also been done on the auditory driving response itself, also known as steady state auditory evoked potentials. Apart from the study by Fredrick et al. (1999), indicating a synchronization effect of auditory stimuli with 18.5Hz repetition rate, most of these studies work with stimuli repetition rates in the gamma range from 30 to 50Hz (Galambos, Makeig, & Talmachoff, 1981; Stapells, Linden, Suffield, Hamel, & Picton, 1984; Linden, Campbell, Hamel, & Picton, 1985; Rees, Green, & Kay, 1986, Jerger, Chmiel, Frost, & Coker, 1986; Picton, Vajsar, Rodriguez, & Campbell, 1987; Galambos & Makeig, 1988; Makeig & Galambos, 1989a, 1989b; Makeig, 1990; Galambos, 1992). Gamma band responses in humans are time-locked to the stimuli with a tightly time-locked as well as a more variable component (Galambos, 1992; Snyder & Large, 2005), and have a relatively short latency (< 50ms; Galambos et al., 1981; Galambos & Makeig, 1988). Başar-Eroglu and Başar (1991) have demonstrated that in cats, visual and auditory stimuli evoke gamma responses in various brain regions. Induced, evoked as well as emitted gamma responses to visual and auditory stimuli have been described.

The latter are bursts of gamma band oscillations time locked to a stimulus (a series of stimuli) that has been omitted; they are thought to reflect stimulus anticipation or expectation on the basis of a postulated timing system that predicts future events (Başar-Eroglu & Başar, 1991). Interestingly, in a clinical study on sensory processing in schizophrenic patients, investigators found that the inability to entrain to gamma frequency auditory clicks, in the manner described above, is a reliable indicator of schizophrenia (Kwon, 1999).

Auditory steady state responses reach a response maximum at stimulation rates around 40Hz (Galambos et al., 1981) and three types of modulations of the response have been identified (Galambos & Makeig, 1988):

spontaneous (circa minute-scale fluctuations), sleep-related (amplitude drops of 50% in sleep states), and stimulus related modulations. A special class of stimulus related modulations, the CERPs or complex event related potentials, lasting for about 400–500 ms, was identified following intensity or frequency changes in the stimulus sequence (Makeig & Galambos, 1989a, 1989b).

Effects of slower frequency stimulation (beta [13–30Hz], alpha [8–12Hz], theta [4–8], and delta [1–4]) have also been reported, but need much more study. Effects in this range are interesting given the fact that most rhythms in music have event durations between 1,000 and 62.5 ms (below the lower threshold events begin to blend into one another). However, from an entrainment perspective it seems important to make a clear distinction between the event (note/tone) durations in a rhythmical figure and the tempo (pulse or beat) of the music: *It is the regular aspect of music that entrains, not the irregular, constantly changing one (though the latter can play a significant role in drawing attention, signaling, etc.).* The lack of studies with stimulus repetition rates up to 4 or 5 events per second comes as a special surprise in view of the overwhelming evidence for an optimal tempo of human repetitive perceptuomotor behavior. Pulse (or beat) tempi that fall roughly between 0.5 and 4Hz are preferred for listening to and making music, result in maximal accuracy in detecting deviant event interval durations, produce the highest accuracy in tapping synchronization experiments, and have been proven similarly optimal in other areas (Van Noorden & Moelants, 1999; Drake, Jones, & Baruch, 2000).

In a review, Lawrence Ward (2003, p. 557) discussed findings on alpha wave synchronization in the context of an oscillatory model of attention originated by Large and Jones (1999):

> Attentional effort, or resource, is assumed to occur in oscillatory pulses, distributed in time by a simple phase oscillator whose period and phase can be entrained by rhythmical external stimuli such as music. When not entrained the phase and period drift around, possibly at an average frequency of 0.5 to 2Hz, and the focus widens. In the presence of external rhythmical stimuli, however, period and phase become entrained to the rhythm, and focus narrows to the emphasized points in time. The consequence of this focus on specific time points is that *stimuli that occur when expected are processed more effectively*, whereas those that occur at unexpected times suffer processing deficits. Importantly, under such conditions alpha oscillations are phase-locked to the occurrences of the entraining stimuli, even when they are omitted, indicating that attentional resources are being mustered for those specific processing moments. (italics added by editors)

Alpha frequency synchronization (with possible entrainment) has also been reported in a study on complex rhythmic music in which the subjects listened to a Mozart symphony and chanting (Rogers & Walter, 1981). This response was compared to their response to non-rhythmic conversation. The study reports increased alpha power during the rhythmic conditions, and synchronization of the EEG to the stimulus rhythm in the alpha range (around 10Hz). The study did not report any subjective effects of the stimulation.

Neher's 1961 study used drum sounds and repetition rates in the high-delta, theta, and low alpha range.[21] He reported that EEG driving responses can be produced by acoustic stimuli with rates from 3 to 8Hz. The main problem with this study is that Neher was working with direct, non-averaged EEG measurements, and it is not clear whether the identified responses were neurogenic in origin or not. The amplitude of potentials evoked by repetitive auditory stimuli are generally smaller and have a different form than indicated by Neher (see e.g., Goodin, Squires, & Starr, 1978; Näätänen & Picton, 1987; Carver et al., 2002; also see Chapters 2 and 5). However, the fact that he also observed driven (synchronized) responses from the ocular muscles may be seen as an indication for an underlying synchronized neural response. Furthermore, it is possible that the differences in amplitude and waveform find their explanation in the different experimental paradigms applied in these studies (e.g., continuous versus intermittent stimulation). Although not much is known about differences in waveform response to continuous and intermittent stimulation, Chapter 5 of this volume presents some of the features that characterize these different responses.

NOTES

1. See One Sound: Traditional Buddhist Music From Tibet, China, Vietnam, Korea, Sri Lanka, and Japan. Audio Disc. Ellipsis Arts, 2000.
2. Rouget, p. 175.
3. Needham, 1967, pp. 606–614.
4. Needham, 1967, pp. 606–614.
5. Sturtevant, 1968, p. 133.
6. Sturtevant, 1968, p. 134.
7. Walker, 1985, p. 172.
8. Walker, 1985, p. 172.
9. Rouget, 1985, p. 172.
10. For more on this, see Chapter 5 of this volume.
11. Jones, 1976, p. 340.
12. Bernieri et al., 1988, p. 244.
13. Jones & Boltz, 1989.
14. Jones & Boltz, 1989.
15. Personal communication with Robert Kauffman, 2005.
16. See Becker's contribution in Chapter 3 of this volume.
17. See Tomaino's overview in Chapter 6.
18. Interestingly, some contributions to this text, especially from Becker (Chapter 3), Jovanov and Maxfield (Chapter 2), Turow and Lane (Chapter 7), and Russell and Turow (Chapter 9), indicate promising directions and possible approaches that eventually might lead to more explicit formulations of a theory of the relationship between rhythm and emotion.

19. For a review see Gruzelier, 1996.
20. See Chapter 9 of this volume.
21. Also see Melinda Maxfield's (1990) study in Chapter 2.

REFERENCES

Adrian, E. D., & Matthews, B. H. C. (1934). The Berger rhythm: potential changes from the occipital lobes in man. *Brain, 57*, 355–384.

Anokhin, A. P., Lutzenberger, W., & Birbaumer, N. (1999). Spatiotemporal organization of brain dynamics and intelligence: An EEG study in adolescents. *The International Journal of Psychophysiology, 33*, 259–273.

Aoki, F., Fetz, E. E., Shupe, L., Lettich, E., & Ojemann, G. A. (1996). Increased gamma-range activity in human sensorimotor cortex during performance of visuomotor tasks. *Clinical Neurophysiology, 110*, 524–537.

Arom, S. (1997). Le syndrome du pentatonism africaine. *Musicae Scienctiae, 1*, 139–163

Baily, J. (2008). Ethnomusicology, intermusability. In H. Strobart (Ed.), *The new (ethno-) musicologies* (pp. 117–134). Lanham, MD: Scarecrow Press.

Bailey Lopez da Silva, F. H. (1991). Neural mechanism underlying brain waves: From neural membranes to networks. *Electroencephalography and Clinical Neurophysiology, 79*, 81–93.

Bailey Lopez da Silva, F. H., & Storm van Leeuwan, W. (1978). The cortical alpha rhythm in dog; the depth and surface profile of phase. In M. A. B. Brazier & H. Petsche (Eds.), *Architectonics of the cerebral cortex* (pp. 319–333). New York: Raven Press.

Barz, G. (2006). *Singing for life: HIV/AIDS and music in Uganda*. New York: Routledge.

Başar, E., Başar-Eroglu, C., Karakas, S., & Schürmann, M. (2000). Brain oscillations in perception and memory. *International Journal of Psychophysiology, 35*, 95–124.

Başar-Eroglu, C., & Başar, E. (1991). A compound P300–40Hz response of the cat hyppocampus. *The International Journal of Neuroscience, 60*, 227–237.

Becker, J. (2001). Anthropological perspectives on music and emotion. In Juslin, P. N. & J. A. Sloboda (Eds.), *Music and emotion* (pp.135–160). Oxford, Oxford University Press.

Berger, H. (1929). Über das Elektrenenkephalogramm des Menschen. *Archive fuer Psychiatrie und Nervenkrankheiten, 87*, 527–570.

Bernardi, L. et al. (2001). BMJ 323 : 1446 doi: 10.1136/bmj.323.7327.1446 (Published 22 December 2001) *British Medical Journal.*

Bernieri, F., Reznick, J. S., & Rosenthal, R. (1988). Synchrony, pseudosynchrony, and dissynchrony: Measuring the entrainment process in mother–infant interactions. *Journal of Personality and Social Psychology, 54*(2), 243–253.

Bittman, B. B., Berk, L. S., Felten, D. L., Westengard, J., Simonton, O. C., Pappas, J., & Ninehouser, M. (2001). Composite effects of group drumming music therapy on modulation of neuroendocrine-immune parameters in normal subjects. *Alternative Therapeutic Health Medicine, 1*, 38–47.

Bittman, B., Bruhn, K. T., Stevens, C., & Westengard, J., & Umbach, P. O. (2003). Recreational music-making: A cost-effective group interdisciplinary strategy for reducing burnout and improving mood states in long-term care workers. *Advanced Mind Body Medicine, 19*(3–4), 16.

Bittman, B. B., Snyder, C., Bruhn, K. T., Liebfreid, F., Stevens, C. K., Westengard, J., & Umbach, P. O. (2004). Recreational music-making: An integrative group intervention for reducing burnout and improving mood states in first year associate degree nursing students: Insights and economic impact. *International Journal of Nursing Education Scholarship, 1*, Article 12. Epub July 9, 2004.

Blacking, J. (1961). Patterns of Nsenga kalimba music. *African Music, 2*, 3–20.

Burgess, A. P., & Gruzelier, J. H. (1997). Short duration synchronization of human theta rhythm during recognition memory. *NeuroReport, 8*, 1039–1042.

Buzsáki, G. (2006). *Rhythms of the brain*. New York: Oxford University Press.

Carter, J. L., & Russell, H. L. (1993). A pilot investigation of auditory and visual entrainment of brain wave activity in learning disabled boys. *Texas Researcher, 4*, 65–73.

Carver, F. W., Fuchs, A., Jantzen, K.J., Kelso, J. A. S. (2002). Spatiotemporal analysis oft he neuromagnetic response to rhythmic auditory stimulation: rate dependence and transient to steady-state transition. *Clinical Neurophysiology, 113*, 1921–1931.

Clayton, M. R., Sager, R., & Will, U. (2005). In time with the music: The concept of entrainment and its significance for ethnomusicology. *European Meetings in Ethnomusicology, 11*, 3–75.

Condon, W. S. (1975). Multiple response to sound in dysfunctional children. *Journal of Autism and Childhood Schizophrenia, 5*(1) 43.

Cooper, R., Winter, A., Crow, H., & Walter, W. G. (1965). Comparison of subcortical, cortical, and scalp activity using chronically indwelling electrodes in man. *Electroencephalography and Clinical Neurophysiology, 18*, 217–230.

Coull, B. M., & Pedley, T. A. (1978). Intermittent photic stimulation. Clinical usefulness of non-conclusive responses. *Electroencephalography and Clinical Neurophysiology, 44*, 353–363.

Cross, I. (2003). Music as biocultural phenomenon. *Annals of the New York Academy of Sciences, 999*, 106–111.

Dieter, J. N. I., & Weinstein, J. A. (1995). The effects of variable frequency photostimulation goggles on EEG and subjective conscious state. *Journal of Mental Imagery, 19*, 77–90.

Drake, C., Jones, M. R., & Baruch, C. (2000). The development of rhythmic attending in auditory sequences: Attunement, referent period, focal attending. *Cognition, 77*, 251–288.

Duffy, F. H., Iyer, V. G., & Surwillo, W. W. (1989). *Clinical and electroencephalography and topographic brain mapping*. New York: Spinger-Verlag.

Eckhorn, R., Bauer, R., Jordan, W., Brosch, M., Kruse, W., Munk, M., & Reitboeck, H. J. (1988). Coherent oscillations: A mechanism of feature linking in the visual cortex? Multiple electrode and correlation analyses in the cat. *Biological Cybernetics, 60*, 121–130.

Eliade, M. (1964). *Shamanism: Archaic techniques of ecstasy*. Princeton, NJ: Princeton University Press. [Table of Contents].

Engel, A. K., Konig, P., Kreiter, A. K., & Singer, W. (1991). Interhemispheric synchronization of oscillatory neuronal responses in cat visual cortex. *Nature, 252*, 1177–1179.

Evans, J. R., & Park, N. S. (1996). Quantitative EEG abnormalities in a sample of dyslexic persons. *Journal of Neurotherapy, 2*(1), 1–5.

Frederick, J. A., Lubar, J. F., Rasey, H. W., Brim, S. A., & Blackburn, J. (1999). Effects of 18.5Hz auditory and visual stimulation on EEG amplitude at the vertex. *Journal of Neurotherapy, 3*, 23–27.

Freeman, W. (1995). *Society of brains: A study in the neuroscience of love and hate*. Hillsdale, NJ: Lawrence Erlbaum Associates.

Friedman, R. (2001, April). Drumming for health. *Percussive Notes*, 55–57.

Galambos, R. (1992). A comparison of certain gamma band (40Hz) brain rhythms in cat and man. In E. Basar & T. H. Bullock (Eds.), *Induced rhythms in the brain* (pp. 201–216). Boston, Basel, Berlin: Birkhuser.

Galambos, R., & Makeig, S. (1988). Dynamic changes in steady state potentials. In E. Basar (Ed.), *Dynamics of sensory and cognitive processing of the brain* (pp. 102–122). Berlin, Heidelberg, New York: Springer.

Galambos, R., Makeig, S., & Talmachoff, P. (1981). A 40Hz auditory potential recorded from the human scalp. *Proceedings of the National Academy of Sciences, USA, 78*(40), 2643–2647.

Gavalas, R. J., Walter, D. O., Hamer, J., & Adey, W. R. (1970). Effects of low-level, low-frequency electric fields on EEG and behavior in Macaca uemestriua. *Brain Research, 18*, 491–501.

Goldman, J. (2004). *Sonic entrainment.* IV International Music-Medicine Symposium, 1989, at Rancho Mirage, CA. Retrieved March 17, 2004 from http://www.healingsounds.com/articles/sonic-entrainment.asp

Goodin, D. S., Squires, K. C., & Starr, A. (1978). Long latency event-related components of the auditory evoked potentials in dementia. *Brain, 101*, 635–648.

Gray, C. M., & Viana Di Prisco, G. (1997). Stimulus-dependent neuronal oscillations and local synchronization in striate cortex of the alert cat. *Journal of Neuroscience, 17*(9), 3239–3253.

Gruzelier, J. H. (1996). New advances in EEG and cognition. International *Journal of Psychophysiology, 24*, 1–5.

Haas, F., Distenfeld, S., & Axen, K. (1986). Effects of perceived musical rhythm on respiratory pattern. *Journal of Applied Physiology, 61*(3), 1185–1191.

Hoffman, D. A., Stockdale, S., Hicks, L. L., & Schwaninger, B. A. (1995). Diagnosis and treatment of head injury. *Journal of Neurotherapy, 1*(1), 14–21.

Isaichev, S. A., Derevyankin, V. T., Koptelov, Yu. M., & Sokolov, E. N. (2001). Rhythmic alpha-activity generators in the human EEG. *Neuroscience and Behavioral Physiology, 31*(1), 49–53.

Jackson, A. (1968) Sound and ritual. *Man, 3*, 293–299.

Jackson, M. (1989). *Paths towards a clearing: Radical empiricism and ethnographic inquiry.* Bloomington: Indiana University Press.

Janowiak, J. J., & Hackman, R. (1994). Meditation and college students' self-actualization and rated stress. *Psychological Reports, 75*(2), 1007–1010.

Jerger, J. F., Chmiel, R., Frost, J. D., & Coker, N. (1986). Effect of sleep on the auditory steady state evoked potential. *Ear Hear, 7*(4), 240–245.

Jones, M. R. (1976). Time, our lost dimension: Toward a new theory of perception, attention, and memory. *Psychological Review, 83*(5), 323–355.

Jones, M. R., & Boltz, M. (1989). Dynamic attending and responses to time. *Psychological Review, 96*(3), 459–491.

Joyce, M., & Siever, D. (2000). Audio-Visual Entrainment (AVE) program as a treatment for behavior disorders in a school setting. *The Journal of Neurotherapy, 4*(2), 9–25.

Keil, A., Muller, M. M., Ray, W. J., Gruber, T., & Elbert, T. (1999). Human gamma band activity and perception of a gestalt. *Journal of Neuroscience, 19*, 7152–7161.

Keil, C. (1998). Applied sociomusicology and performance studies. *Ethno-musicology, 42*(2), 303 ff.

Keil, C., & Feld, S. (1994). *Music grooves.* Chicago: University of Chicago Press.

Klimesch, W. (1999). EEG alpha and theta oscillations reflect cognitive and memory performance: A review and analysis. *Brain Research Reviews, 29*, 169–195.

Klimesch, W., Schimke, H., & Schwaiger, J. (1994). Episodic and semantic memory: An analysis in the EEG theta and alpha band. *Electroencephalography and Clinical Neurophysiology, 91*, 428–441.

Koen, B. D. (Ed.). (2008). *The Oxford handbook of medical ethnomusicology.* Oxford University Press.

Kwon, J. S., O'Donnell, B. F., Wallenstein, G. V., Greene, R. W., Hirayasu, Y., Nestor, P. G., . . . McCarley, R. W. (1999). Gamma frequency-range abnormalities to auditory stimulation in schizophrenia. *Archives of General Psychiatry, 56*(11), 1001–1005.

Labby, D. (1976). *The demystification of yap.* Chicago: University of Chicago Press.

Large, E. W., & Jones, M. R. (1999). The dynamics of attending: How people track time-varying events. *Psychological Review, 106,* 119–159.

Large, E. W., & Kolen, J. F. (1994). Resonance and the perception of musical meter. *Connection Science: Journal of Neural Computing, Artificial Intelligence and Cognitive Research, 6*(2–3), 177–208.

Lee, M. S., Bae, B. H., Ryu, H., Sohn, J. H., Kim, S. Y., & Chung, H. T. (1997). Changes in alpha wave and state anxiety during ChunDoSunBup Qi-training in trainees with open eyes. *American Journal of Chinese Medicine, 25*(3–4), 289–299.

Linden, R. D., Campbell, K. B, Hamel, G., & Picton, T. (1985). Human auditory steady state evoked potentials during sleep. *Ear Hear, 6,* 167–174.

Makeig, S. (1990). A dramatic increase in the auditory middle latency response at very slow rates. In C. M. Brunia, A. K. Gaillard, & A. Kok (Eds.), *Psychological brain research* (pp. 56–60). Tillburg, the Netherlands: Tillburg University Press.

Makeig, S., & Galambos, R. (1989a). The auditory 40Hz-band evoked response lasts 150 ms and increases in size at slow rates. *Society for Neuroscience Abstracts, 15,* 113.

Makeig, S., & Galambos, R. (1989b). The CERP: Event-related perturbations in steady state responses. In E. Basar & T. H. Bullock (Eds.), *Brain dynamics: Progress and perspectives* (pp. 375–400). Berlin: Springer.

Maltseva, I., et al. (2000). Alpha oscillations as an indicator of dynamic memory operations: Anticipation of omitted stimuli. *International Journal of Psychophysiology, 36,* 185–197.

Mandell, A. (1980). Toward a psychobiology of transcendence: God in the brain. In D. Davidson & R. Davidson (Eds.), *The psychobiology of consciousness* (pp. 379–464). New York: Plenum Press.

Maurer, R. L., Sr., Kumar, V. K., Woodside, L., & Pekala, R. J. (1997). Phenomenological experience in response to monotonous drumming and hypnotizability. *American Journal of Clinical Hypnosis, 40*(2), 130–145.

McAuley, D., Jones, M. R., Holub, Sh., Johnston, H. M., & Miller, N. S. (2006). The time of our lives: Life span development of timing and event tracking. *Journal of Experimental Psychology: General, 135*(3), 348–367.

McIntosh, G.C., Thaut, M.H., & Rice, R.R. 1996. Rhythmic auditory stimulation as entrainment and therapy technique in gait of stroke and Parkinson's disease patients. In R. Pratt & R. Spintge (Eds.), *Music Medicine*, Vol. II (pp. 145–152). St. Louis, MO: MMB Music.

Merker, B. (1999). Synchronous chorusing and the origins of music. In C. Trevarthen (Ed.), *Rhythm, musical narrative, and origins of musical communication.* Special issue of *Musicae Scientiae* (pp. 59–73).

Micheletti, L. (1999). *The use of light and sound stimulation for the treatment of attention deficit hyperactivity disorder in children.* Dissertation, University of Texas, Houston.

Miltner, W. H. R., Braun, C., Arnold, M., Witte, M., & Taub, E. (1999). Coherence of gamma-band EEG activity as a basis for associative learning. *Nature, 397,* 434–436.

Montgomery, D. D., Ashley, E., Burns, W. J., & Russell, H. L. (1994). Clinical outcome of a single case study of EEG entrainment for closed head injury. *Proceedings from the Association for Applied Psychophysiology and Biofeedback*, *25*, 82–83.

Morse, D. R. (1993). Brain wave synchronizers: A review of their stress reduction effects and clinical studies assessed by questionnaire, galvanic skin resistance, pulse rate, saliva, and electroencephalograph. *Stress Medicine, 9*, 111–126.

Mueller, H. H., Donaldson, C. C. S., Nelson, D. V., & Layman, M. (2001). Treatment of fibromyalgia incorporating EEG-driven stimulation. *Journal of Clinical Psychology, 57*(7), 933–952.

Muller, M. M., Bosch, J., Elbert, T., Kreiter, A., Sosa, M. V., Sosa, P. V., & Rockstroh, B. (1996). Visually induced gamma-band responses in human electroencephalographic activity. A link to animal studies. *Experimental Brain Research, 112*, 96–102.

Näätänen, R. and Picton, T. W. (1987) & Picton, T. (1987). The N1 wave of the human electric and magnetic response to sound: A review and an analysis of the component structure. *Psychphysiology*, 24(4), 375–425.

Namerow, N. S., Sclabassi, R. J., & Enns, N. F. (1974). Somatosensory responses to stimulus trains: Normative data. *Electroencephalography and Clinical Neurophysiology, 37*, 11–21.

Néda, Z., Ravasz, E., Brechet, Y., Vicsek, T., & Barabsi, A. L. (2000). Self-organizing process: The sound of many hands clapping. *Nature, 403*, 849–850.

Neher, A. (1961). Auditory driving observed with scalp electrodes in normal subjects. *Electroencephalography and Clinical Neurophysiology, 13*, 449–451.

Neher, A. (1962). A physiological explanation of unusual behavior in ceremonies involving drums. *Human Biology, IV*, 151–160.

Noton, D. (1997). PMS, EEG, and photic stimulation. *Journal of Neurotherapy, 2*(2), 8–13.

Nunez, R. (1997). Eatring soup with chopsticks: Dogmas, difficulties, and alternatives in the study of conscious experience. *Journal of Consciousness Studies, 4*(2), 143–166.

Octravia, I., Luis, H., & Antunes, J. (2005). The physics of Tibetan singing bowls. *Revista de Acoustica, 35*, 33–39.

Picton, T. W., Vajsar, J., Rodriguez, R., & Campbell, K. B. (1987). Reliability estimates for steady-state evoked potentials. *Electroencephalography and Clinical Neurophysiology, 68*, 119–131.

Pikovsky, A., Rosenblum, M., & Kurths, J. (2001). *Synchronization. A universal concept in nonlinear science.* Cambridge, UK: Cambridge University Press.

Pollock, V. E., Volavka, J., Gabrielli, W. F., Grings, W. W., Stern, & J. A. (1986). Brain responses to sine wave modulated light (SML): Reliability and relationship to spontaneous EEG. *International Journal of Neuroscience, 29*(3–4), 255–263.

Pompeiano, O., & Swett, J. E. (1962). EEG and behavioral manifestations of sleep induced by cutaneous nerve stimulation in normal cats. *Archives Italiennes de Biologie, 100*, 311–342.

Rees, A., Green, G. G. R., & Kay, R. H. (1986). Steady-state evoked responses to sinusoidally amplitude-modulated sound recorded in man. *Hearing Research, 23*, 123–133.

Rodriguez, E., George, N., Lachaux, J., Martinerie, J., Renault, B., & Varela, F. (1999). Perceptions shadow: Long-distance synchronization of human brain activity. *Nature, 397*, 430–433.

Rogers, L. J., & Walter, D. O. (1981). Methods for finding single generators, with application to auditory driving of the human EEG by complex stimuli. *Journal of Neuroscience Methods, 4*(3), 257–265.

Rouget, G. (1985). *Music and trance: A theory of the relations between music and possession.* Chicago: University of Chicago Press.

Rozelle, G. R., & Budzynski, T. H. (1995). Neurotherapy for stroke rehabilitation: A single case study. *Biofeedback Self-Regulation, 20*(3), 211–228.

Russell, H. L. (1997). Intellectual, auditory, and photic stimulation and changes in functioning in children and adults. *Biofeedback, 25*(1), 16–17, 23–24.

Safranek, M., Koshland, G., & Raymond, G. (1982). Effect of auditory rhythm on muscle activity. *Physical Therapy, 62,* 161–168.

Seer, P., & Raeburn, J. M. (1980). Meditation training and essential hypertension: A methodological study. *Journal of Behavioral Medicine, 3*(1), 59–71.

Silberstein, R. B. (1995). Neuromodulation of neocortical dynamics. In P. L. Nunez (Ed.), *Neocortical dynamics and human EEG rhythms* (pp. 591–627). New York: Oxford University Press.

Snyder, J. S., & Large, E. W. (2005). Gamma-band activity reflects the metric structure of rhythmic tone sequences. *Cognitive Brain Research, 24,* 117–126.

Solomon, G. D. (1985). Slow wave photic stimulation in the treatment of headache—a preliminary study. *Headache, 25,* 444–446.

Stapells, D. R., Linden, R. D., Suffield, J. B., Hamel, G., & Picton, T. W. (1984). Human auditory steady state potentials. *Ear Hear, 5*(2), 105–114.

Stigsby, B., Rodenberg, J. C., & Moth, H. B. (1981). Electroencephalographic findings during mantra meditation (transcendental meditation). A controlled, quantitative study of experienced meditators. *Electroencephalography and Clinical Neurophysiology, 51*(4), 434–442.

Strathern, M. (1992). *After nature: English kinship in the late twentieth century.* Cambridge: Cambridge University Press.

Strobart, H. (Ed.). (2008). *The new (ethno-) musicologies.* Lanham, MD: Scarcrow Press.

Strogatz, S. (2003). *Sync, the emerging science of spontaneous order.* New York: Hyperion.

Szabó, C. (2004). The effects of monotonous drumming on subjective experiences. *Music Therapy Today,* V(1), pp. 1–9.

Takahashi, T. (1987). Activation methods. In E. Niedermeyer, F. Lopez da Silva (Eds.), *Electroencephalography, basic principles, clinical applications and related fields, ed. 2* (pp. 209–227). Baltimore: Urban and Scharzenberg.

Tallon, C., Bertrand, O., Bouchet, P., & Pernier, J. (1995). Gamma-range activity evoked by coherent visual stimuli in humans. *European Journal of Neuroscience, 7,* 1285–1291.

Tallon-Baudry, C., Bertrand, O., & Fischer, C. (2001). Oscillatory synchrony between human extrastriate areas during visual short-term memory maintenance. *Journal of Neuroscience, 21*(15), RC177.

Thaut, M. H., McIntosh, G. C., Prassas, S. G., & Rice, R. R. (1992). Effect of rhythmic cuing on temporal stride parameters and EMG patterns in normal gait. *Journal of Neurologic Rehabilitation, 6,* 185–190.

Thaut, M. H., McIntosh, G. C., Prassas, S. G., & Rice, R. R. (1993). Effect of rhythmic cuing on temporal stride parameters and EMG patterns in hemiparetic stroke patients. *Journal of Neurologic Rehabilitation, 7,* 9–16.

Thaut, M.H., Schleiffers, S., & Davis, W.B. 1992. Changes in EMG patterns under the influence of auditory rhythm. In R. Spintge & R. Droh (Eds.), Music Medicine (pp. 80–101). St. Louis (MO): MMB Music.

Timmerman, D., Lubar, J. F., Rasey, H. W., & Frederick, J. A. (1999). Effects of dominant and twice-dominant alpha audiovisual stimulation on the cortical EEG. *International Journal of Psychophysiology, 32,* 55–61.

Toman, J. (1941). Flicker potentials and the alpha rhythm in man. *Journal of Neurophysiology, 4*, 51–61.

Townsend, R. E., Lubin, A., & Naitoh, P. (1975). Stabilization of alpha frequency by sinusoidally modulated light. *Electroencephalography and Clinical Neurophysiology, 39*, 515–518.

Trevarthen, C. (1999). Musicality and the intrinsic motive pulse: Evidence from human psychobiology and infant communication. In C. Trevarthen (Ed.), *Rhythm, musical narrative, and origins of musical communication* (pp. 155–215). Special issue of *Musicae Scientiae*.

Turner, V. (1987). Body, brain, and culture. In V. Turner, *The anthropology of performance*. New York: PAJ Publications.

Van Noorden, L., & Moelants, D. (1999). Resonance in the perception of musical pulse. *Journal of New Music Research, 28*(1), 43–66.

Varela, F. J. (1988). Structural coupling and the origin of meaning in simple cellular automata. In E. Secarz, F. Celada, N. A. Mitchinson, & T. Tada (Eds.), *The semiotics of cellular communication in the immune system*. New York: Springer, pp. 151–161).

Varela, F. J., Thompson, E., & Rosch, E. (1991). *The embodied mind*. Cambridge, MA: MIT Press.

Wachiuli, M., Koyama, M., Utsuyama, M., Bittman, B. B., Kitagawa, M., & Hirokawa, K. (2007). Recreational music-making modulates natural killer cell activity, cytokines, and mood states in corporate employees. *Medical Science Monitor, 13*(2), CR57–70.

Wada, Y., Nanbu, Y., Kadoshima, R., & Jiang, Z. Y. (1996). Interhemispheric EEG coherence during photic stimulation: Sex differences in normal young adults. *International Journal of Psychophysiology, 22*(1–2), 45–51.

Wada, Y., Nanbu, Y., Kikuchi, M., Koshino, Y., & Hashimoto, T. (1998). Aberrant functional organization in schizophrenia: Analysis of EEG coherence during rest and photic stimulation in drug-naive patients. *Neuropsychobiology, 38*(2), 63–69.

Wada, Y., Nanbu, Y., Kikuchi, M., Koshino, Y., Hashimoto, T., & Yamaguchi, N. (1998). Abnormal functional connectivity in Alzheimer's disease: Intrahemispheric EEG coherence during rest and photic stimulation. *European Archives of Psychiatry and Clinical Neuroscience, 248*(4), 203–208.

Walker, S. S. (1972). Ceremonial spirit possession in Africa and Afro-America (pp. 17–24). Leiden: EJ. Brill.

Walter, D. O., & Adey, W. R. (1966). Linear and nonlinear mechanisms of brainwave generation. *Annals of the New York Academy of Sciences, 128*, 772–780.

Walter, W. G. (1953). *The living brain*. New York: Norton.

Walter, W. G., Dovey, V. J., & Shipton, H. (1946). Analysis of electrical response of human cortex to photic stimulation. *Nature, 158*, 340–541.

Walton, K., & Levitsky, D. (1994). A neuroendocrine mechanism for the reduction of drug use and addictions by transcendental meditation. In D. O'Connell & C. Alexander (Eds.), *Self-recovery: Treating addictions using transcendental meditation and Maharishi Ayur-Veda Press* (pp. 89–117). New York: Haworth.

Ward, L. M. (2002). Synchronous relaxation oscillators and inner psychophysics. In J. A. Da Silva, et al., (Eds.), Fechner day (pp. 145–150). *International Society for Psychophysics*.

Ward, L. M. (2003). Synchronous neural oscillations and cognitive processes. *Trends in Cognitive Sciences, 7*(12), 553–559.

Widdess, R., Will, U., & Clayton, M. R. (2005). *Analytical approaches to unmetered rhythm: Case studies of North Indian alap*. Panel presentation at the 50th Annual Meeting of the Society for Ethnomusicology, Atlanta, GA, October.

Wiener, N. (1958). *Non-linear problems in random theory*. MIT Press: Cambridge, MA.

Will, U. (1999). La baguette magique dethnomusicologie. Re- penser la no-tation et lanalyse de la musique.(The magic wand of ethnomusicology. Re-thinking notation and its application in music analyses) In G. Georg, *Cahiers de Musiques Traditionelles*, Vol. XII (pp. 9–34), Chêne-Bourg.

Will, U. (2007). In the garden of cultural identities silk flowers quickly grow roots. On the logic of culture race and identity in postmodernist discourse. *European Meetings In Ethnomusicology, 12*, 5–21.

Will, U., & Berg, E. (2007). Brainwave synchronization and entrainment to periodic stimuli. *NeuroScience Letters, 424*, 55–60.

Winkelman, M. (1997). Altered states of consciousness and religious behavior. In S. Glazier (Ed.), *Anthropology of religion: A handbook of method and theory* (pp. 393–428). Westport, CT: Greenwood Press.

Winkelman, M. (2000). *Shamanism: The neural ecology of consciousness and healing*. Westport, CT: Bergin and Garvey.

Winkelman, M. (2003). Complementary therapy for addiction: Drumming out drugs. *The American Journal of Public Health, 93*, 647–651.

Wood, A. (2008). E-fieldwork: A paradigm for the twenty-first century? In H. Strobart (Ed.), *The new (ethno-) musicologies* (p. 170–187). Lanham, MD: Scarcrow Press.

Woodside, L. N., et al. (1997). Monotonous percussion drumming and trance postures: A controlled evaluation of phenomenological effects. *Anthropology of Consciousness, 8*(2–3), 69–87.

2   Entraining the Brain and Body

Emil Jovanov and Melinda C. Maxfield

PART I. EFFECTS OF REPETITIVE RHYTHMIC MUSIC ON EEG AND SUBJECTIVE EXPERIENCE

In 1990, in her interest to explore the posited correlation between drumming tempi and brainwave responses, Melinda Maxfield arranged a lab-based replication of a shamanic drumming ceremony, monitoring subjects' electroencephalographic (EEG) responses while documenting their subjective experiences. Similarly, in 2005, Emil Jovanov completed an exploratory study on experienced yogic meditators, measuring heart rate variability and respiration responses to rhythmic chanting. Both studies, though focused on considerably different traditions, explore the ritual use of rhythmic auditory stimulation as a means to stabilize basic physiological rhythms (breathing, heartbeat, brainwaves) and facilitate altered states of consciousness.

Many oral traditions acknowledge that percussion in general, and rhythmic drumming in particular, facilitates communication with the spiritual world (Crawley, 1912; Rouget, 1985; Eliade, 1964; Needham, 1979; Hart, 1990; Harner, 1990). Shamanic ritual behavior fits this model: In the literature, shamans are most often described as healers, "technicians of the sacred," "masters of ecstasy," who use ritual drumming to deliberately enter into altered states of consciousness to discover information relevant to their patient's ailment and its treatment (Eliade, 1964; Walsh, 1989, 1990; Achterberg, 1985; Drury, 1982, 1989). In shamanic traditions, the drum is often described as a bridge between normal reality and the spirit world. Mircea Eliade, in his seminal work on shamanism, writes: "the shamanic drum is distinguished from all other instruments of the 'magic of noise' precisely by the fact that it makes possible an ecstatic experience" (Eliade, 1964. p. 174). Similarly, Michael Harner, founder of the Foundation for Shamanic Studies, notes: " . . . the repetitive sound of the drum is usually fundamental to undertaking the shamanic task . . . " (Harner, 1990, p. 51).

Despite the relative consensus among ethnomusicologists that drumming is an important catalyst for the shaman's transition into trance (Crawley, 1912; Eliade, 1964; Prince, 1968a, 1968b; Needham, 1979; Rouget, 1985; Hart, 1990; Harner, 1990), the exact relationship between drumming and altered states is not well understood. There is, however, a variety of speculation on the specific role the drum plays in this process. These theories include:

1. Rhythmic drumming acts as a focus for concentration and is used in combination with sensory deprivation, fasting, fatigue, mental imagery, etc., to achieve an altered state of consciousness.
2. Rhythmic drumming is simply part of the "set and setting" dictated by the beliefs and ritualized ceremonies of the culture, and the altered state of consciousness is a product of pathology, trickery, and/or hallucinations stemming from an overactive imagination and hyper-suggestibility.
3. The rhythm of the drumming facilitates an altered state of consciousness.
4. The monotony of the drumming facilitates an altered state of consciousness.
5. The acoustic stimulation of rhythmic drumming acts as an auditory driving mechanism, affecting the electrical activity of the brain by bringing it into resonance (at a particular frequency or set of frequencies) with the external stimuli.

Harner emphasizes this latter theory in his arguments regarding the consistency in shamanic ritual drumming worldwide: It often takes the form of a steady beat, played at 3 to 4 and 1/2 pulses per second, for several hours (Harner, 1990). Neher's (1961) work on auditory driving and dissociation also emphasizes these tempi. Wolfgang Jilek, Emeritus Professor of Psychiatry, University of British Columbia, reports similar findings in his research on the ritual dance drumming of the Salish Indians (Jilek 1974). In this study, Jilek observed a predominance in drumming frequencies at 4 to 7 beats per second, a range that correlates with the theta wave frequency band (4–7Hz) of the human EEG. He hypothesized that stimulation in this frequency range would be the most effective aid to entering an altered state of consciousness, given the correlations between increased theta wave activity and hypnogogic imagery, states of ecstasy, creativity, and sudden illuminations (Achterberg, 1985; Green & Green, 1977).

Brainwaves and Subjective States

As briefly described in Chapter 1, brain electrical activity in various frequency bands is correlated with particular states of consciousness.

- Beta frequency activity (13–30Hz) is associated with active attention and focus on the exterior world, such as normal, everyday activities. Beta is also present during states of tension, anxiety, fear, and alarm (Green & Green, 1977; Spehlmann, 1981; Dyro, 1989).
- Alpha frequency activity (8–13Hz) is most often associated with states of relaxation. Alpha generally appears in the occipital region of the

brain (the visual cortex) when the eyes are closed. In this state, subjects are alert but unfocused, or focused on the interior world (Guyton & Hall, 2006).

- Theta frequency activity (4–8Hz) is usually associated with drowsy, near unconscious states, such as the threshold period just before waking or sleeping. The same activity has often been connected to states of reverie and hypnogogic or dream-like imagery. For most people, it is difficult to maintain consciousness without any outside stimulation during periods of increased theta activity (Tart, 1972; Wallace & Benson, 1972; Banquet, 1973). Research has confirmed that such practices as yoga and meditation produce changes in the electrical activity of the brain that can lead to a baseline increase in alpha and/or theta rhythms (Benson, 1975, p. 82; Murphy & Donovan, 1988). Interestingly, enhanced baseline theta and the maintenance of theta waves during meditation is found to be characteristic of long-term meditators who are able to maintain the theta state while keeping their self-awareness intact (Green & Green, 1986).
- Delta frequency activity (.05–4Hz) is associated with deep sleep or unconsciousness (Guyton & Hall, 2006).

Research

Maxfield's study relied on the biofeedback technology of MindCenter Corporation, formerly located in Palo Alto, CA. This multi-user system was a prototype 16-channel electroencephalographic biofeedback instrument (Grass) running under computer. The channel filters were tuned to broadband theta, alpha, and beta frequencies. The frequencies of the filters band pass zones were: theta, 4–6.7Hz; alpha, 7.7–12.6Hz; beta, 15–24Hz. The multi-user system was composed of four modules, each designed to block external sound and light. There was no specific temperature control. The participants were able to lie down inside the module in the traditional drum-journey[1] posture. Each module contained a sound system, consisting of a generic tuner and audio cassette player.

From these modules, four cortical sites were monitored for theta, alpha, and beta brainwave activity. Brainwaves were recorded from each participant on the following cortical sites: left parieto-central, right parieto-central, left parietotemporal, right parieto-temporal. Ground electrodes were placed in the center of the forehead, with reference electrodes for the differential amplifiers on both ears, in linked pairs.

Participants

Twelve subjects, 8 women and 4 men, were selected to participate in the study. The minimum age was 19; the maximum age was 68; the mean age was 39. Eight participants had completed 4 or more years of college, 2 had

Table 2.1   Tape Sequence Schedule

	1:00-4:00 Group A	4:30-7:30 Group B	7:30-10:00 Group C
Monday	I Ching	Free	Shamanic
Wednesday	Free	Shamanic	I Ching
Friday	Shamanic	I Ching	Free

completed 2 or more years of college, and 2 had completed, or were in the process of completing, 1 year of college. One of the main criterions for subject selection was limited experience with rhythmic drumming patterns and a lack of general knowledge regarding shamanic rituals. Additionally, no one with a history of psychosis, epilepsy, and/or other neurophysiological disorders was accepted to participate.

Psychological Testing Instruments

Four weeks prior to the first session, each participant completed a battery of mood scale tests (Dean J. Clyde Mood Scale [Clyde], Multiple Affect Adjective Check List [MAACL], Profile of Mood States [POMS]). These scales were mailed to participants in their initial information packet. The mood scale tests were administered again before and after each session. These results are not included here, but subjects' subjective reports are summarized below.

The 12 participants were divided into 3 groups of 4. Each group was tested in 3 sessions, on 3 separate days, for a total of 36 individual sessions. (The actual total of individual sessions was 35, as 1 participant canceled a session due to a work-related crisis.) Group A was in the laboratory from 1 to 4 p.m., Group B from 4:30 to 7:30 p.m., and Group C from 7:30 to 10:30 p.m. on Monday, Wednesday, and Friday during the testing week. Each group was exposed to three drumming tapes, one tape per day. Participants were monitored for EEG responses to each of the three tapes; the tapes were counter-balanced for each group during each session to control for order effects. In lieu of live drumming in the lab, four drummers were hired to record the experiment tapes in a local commercial sound studio. Each 20-minute tape featured one kind of drumming:

1. *Shamanic Drumming:* the type of "core" shamanic drumming journey described and popularized by Harner (1990), with sustained, monotonous beats in unison, ranging from approximately 4 to 4.5 beats per second (Hz), or 240–270 beats per minute (BPM).

2. *I Ching Drumming:* a rhythmic, syncopated drumming pattern, ranging from approximately 3 to 4Hz (180–240 BPM), inspired by (I
   Ching, 1950).
3. *Free Drumming:* incorporates no sustained rhythmic pattern.

Session Details

1. Upon their arrival at the laboratory, participants were fitted with
   electrodes.
2. The participants were escorted to the modules to which they had been
   assigned for the three sessions. Mood scale tests (MAACL, Clyde,
   and POMS) were administered via the computer contained in the
   module.
3. Upon completion of the mood tests, the participants were placed in a
   prone position on the module floor. Foam pads and pillows were provided for comfort. A technician connected the scalp electrode wires
   to the appropriate terminals. The module was then closed. Communication with the participants was accomplished through the module
   intercom system.
4. Participants were instructed by the technician to relax with eyes
   closed and to restrict body movements.
5. Baseline theta, alpha, and beta were taken, including and in the following order:
   - 4 minutes of baseline with eyes open;
   - 8 minutes of baseline with eyes closed;
   - 8 minutes of baseline with white noise (eyes closed).
6. A drumming tape was then played through the modules sound system
   for 20 minutes.
7. When the drumming tape ended, more baselines were taken, including: 8 minutes of white noise, 8 minutes eyes closed, and 4 minutes
   eyes open baselines.
8. The modules were opened. The technicians detached the electrode
   wires from the module connection so that the participants could sit
   in a chair to work the computer keyboard. Mood scales were again
   administered via the computer in the module.
9. Participants left the modules and were taken to a room where they
   were asked to give a brief written account of their subjective experience. Most were able to accomplish this task within 15 to 20 minutes. Art supplies were available for those who wished to capture their
   memories through drawing and color.
10. Participants were then given an interview (10 to 15 minutes) by the author
    in which they gave an oral summary of their experience. This interview
    was tape-recorded. These subjective experiences were then categorized
    according to recurring themes and consensual topics. Those who had

completed their written account and were waiting for an interview, used the time to allow the technicians to remove the scalp electrodes.

None of the participants were given information on imaging and/or the shamanic journey, and all had previously given assurance that they were naive to the details and the experience of shamanic journeying in the context of rhythmic drumming. After data collection was completed, movement artifacts were eliminated from the EEG record and corresponding digital printouts.

Results

Data were derived from wave amplitudes integrated during 15-second epochs to represent total EEG band power in theta, alpha, and beta from each site. Baseline scores were printed out every 15 seconds during the three-part baseline procedures. Scores during the drumming session were printed out every 2 minutes. In order to condense and interpret the sizeable amount of data obtained from these procedures, epochs were selected for analysis at 2, 9, 13, 15, and 20 minutes. These times were selected because:

- Sampling at 2 minutes would represent the state of subjects' brainwaves after initial settling in;
- Sampling at 9, 13, 15 minutes would record subjects optimum physiological response to drumming;[2]
- ampling at 20 minutes was used to determine final changes in frequency band power relative to baselines, and relative to previous epochs.

Absolute means on each time epoch for theta, alpha, and beta brainwave patterns, recorded at each of the four cortical sites, yielded a total of 72 per person per session, or a total of 2,592 absolute means. Mean difference scores (MDS) were obtained by subtracting each individual's absolute mean scores (obtained during the beginning white noise baseline) from every score for the five time epochs, the four cortical sites, and the three brainwave patterns, yielding a total of 2,160 MDS.

Example: Subject 1A (left temporal activity)
Theta absolute mean score baseline = +159
Theta absolute mean score for minute 2 during Shamanic Drumming
    = -135
Mean difference score = -24

This technique corrects somewhat for individual differences in EEG band power. Baselines were derived from the beginning white noise segments. As was normal protocol in this particular lab, the white noise incorporated random beeps that the participant was asked to count in order to reveal a picture of normal brain activity in a baseline alert state.

Group Means Differences (MDS) for Total Theta, Alpha, and Beta for Three Drumming Patterns

Group mean differences from baseline scores were derived for total theta, alpha,and beta (averaged for each of the four cortical sites), for minutes 2, 9, 13, 15, and 20 for each of the three drumming patterns. Two sets of graphs are presented: In the first set (Figure 2.1, Figure 2.2, and Figure 2.3), group means scores for total theta, alpha, and beta are shown. A separate graph is provided for each drumming pattern. In the second set

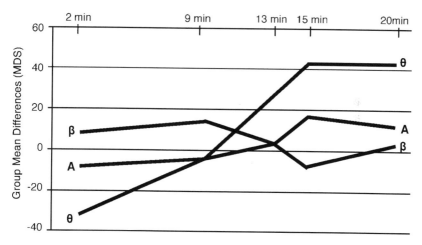

Figure 2.1 Group mean differences (MDS) for total theta, alpha, and beta for shamanic drumming.

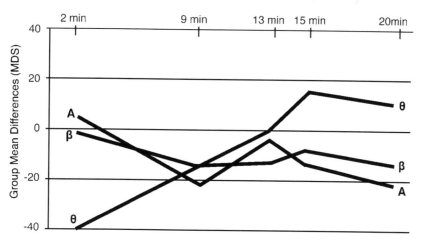

Figure 2.2 Group mean differences (MDS) for total theta, alpha, and beta for I Ching drumming.

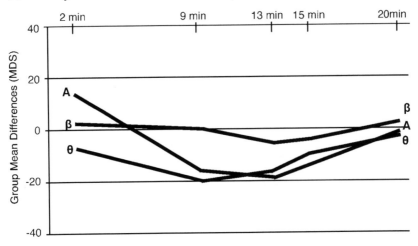

Figure 2.3   Group mean differences (MDS) for total theta, alpha, and beta for free drumming.

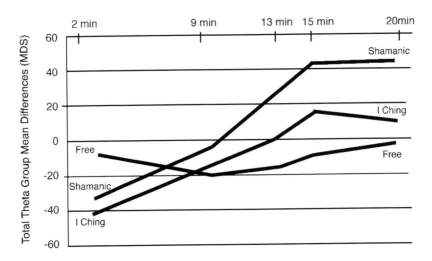

Figure 2.4   Total theta group mean differences (MDS) for the three drumming patterns.

(Figure 2.4, Figure 2.5, and Figure 2.6), a separate graph is provided for each brainwave frequency (theta, alpha, and beta).

The greatest response is seen during the Shamanic Drumming, which shows increased theta band power (Figure 2.1). The greatest response was measured from the right temporal lead, with a rapid rise to minute 15. The greatest gain in alpha is seen during Shamanic Drumming in the left

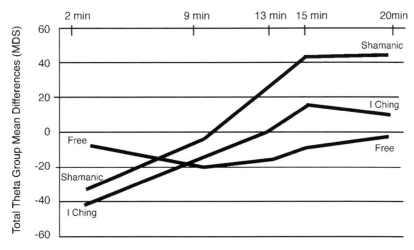

Figure 2.5 Total beta group mean differences (MDS) for the three drumming patterns.

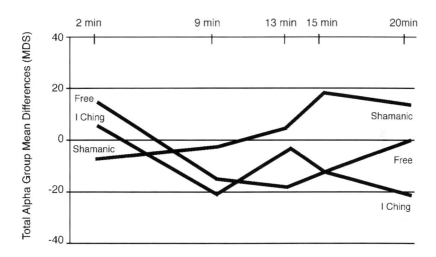

Figure 2.6 Total alpha group mean differences (MDS) for the three drumming patterns.

hemisphere, peaking at minute 15. A lesser increase in theta is found during the I Ching Drumming (Figure 2.2), peaking at minute 15; similarly, the greatest response was measured in the right temporal region. Brain-wave activity for all three frequency bands appeared to remain constant or decline during Free Drumming (Figure 2.3). There was no significant gain in beta band power from any drumming pattern.

It is interesting to note that all 12 participants had visual and/or somatic imagery during stimulation. For 8 of these 12, the images were dreamlike, but vivid. The following short examples typify their accounts:

Subject A:

"Immediately, I saw a heart pumping to the beat of the drums. There were two drum beats to every heartbeat. . . . I saw an African dance, at night, with big drums and dancers in costumes. I viewed this from a distance." [Maxfield notes:] The subject reported that he was focused on the beat of the drums; the dancing was foggy and in the background. "The auditory beat was the main thing. . . . I was suddenly shot through a tunnel of darkness. I felt the movement up, like being in a channel. I had no clue how I got in it. All of a sudden, I was there. I ended up free in the outer universe. It was dark, but I had a real sense of freedom. It was great. I felt free, excited and relaxed—exhilarated, as if I had let go of something. My body felt a sense of uplifted exhilaration and freedom."

Subject B:

"The drumming emerged as geometric shapes—triangles, squares, and circles. There was lots of color, plus black—very vivid color. The patterns of the sounds went around in vivid colors."

Subject C:

"In the beginning, there was the sense of an Eskimo in a double-headed canoe. . . . Right after the Eskimos, in the beginning, I saw an abstract symbol that became a seal that beckoned me. I joined it and swam through a sea of blue calm. . . . I became a swimming projectile, moving very rapidly. . . . It was a very fast, forward-moving motion. Eventually, I approached a door, which became a series of doors, into the perspective. I went down through a tunnel. My body moved and bent with the tunnel and popped up in another part of the earth. . . . I had many, many, very vivid images. I was right there. . . . Indians, smoke, firelight, mountain lions, prairie-kinds of animals. . . . All of it was 'night-time stuff.' There was no 'daytime stuff' or people. . . . At one point, I saw the opening of a kaleidoscope, round, changing shape and color."

The first 12 categories listed below are the common themes as synthesized from the 12 participants' verbal and written reports of their experiences in one or more sessions during the drumming.
   These include:

- Loss of Time Sense

Seven of the 12 participants stated that they had lost the time continuum, thus having no clear sense of the length of the drumming session.

- Movement Sensations
  Ten of the 12 participants experienced one or more Movement Sensation.
     This category includes the experience of feeling:
     —the body or parts of the body pulsating or expanding;
     —pressure on the body or parts of the body, especially the head, throat, and chest;
     —energy moving in waves through the body; and
     —sensations of flying, spiraling, dancing, running, etc.

- Heightened Arousal
  Nine of the 12 participants mentioned specifically that they became energized during and/or immediately after the drumming session.

- Temperature Fluctuations (Cold/Hot)
  Six of the 12 participants experienced sudden changes in temperature (e.g., chills, being flooded with warmth, sweating.).

- Relaxed, Sharp/Clear
  Five of the 12 participants noticed that they felt particularly relaxed, sharp, and clear. This was usually in lieu of more explicit emotional content.

- Discomfort
  Five of the 12 participants mentioned specifically that they were in varying states of emotional or physical discomfort.

- Journey
  Five of the 12 participants' descriptions of their experiences included classic shamanic journey imagery, such as going into a hole or a cave, being shot through a tube or a tunnel, spiraling up or down, being initiated, climbing an inverted tree, and/or the appearance of power animals and helping allies.

- Images
     —Vivid Imagery: All 12 participants had some imagery. Eight of the 12 commented on experiencing vivid visual or sensate (somatic) images.
     —Natives: Nine of the 12 participants saw or sensed African, Tahi-tian, Eskimo, or Native American natives. These natives were usually participating in rituals and/or ceremonies involving dancing, singing or chanting, hunting, or drumming.

—Animals/Landscapes: Seven of the 12 participants reported a wide range of animal and landscape imagery.

—People: Nine of the 12 participants imaged childhood friends or important people from their past, "faceless" teachers, non-native drummers, unidentified faces.

* Out-of-Body Experiences (OBE) / Visitations
Three of the 12 participants stated that they had the experience of leaving the module or being visited by a presence or a person during the session. This category is differentiated from "Journey" in that no traditional shamanic imagery was present.

* Non-ordinary or altered states of consciousness (ASC)
A majority of the participants, in one or more sessions, were conscious of the fact that there had been a qualitative shift in mental functioning, and the 12 themes as synthesized from the participants' oral and written reports may be correlated with Ludwig's delineation of features that tend to be characteristic of most ASCs (Ludwig, 1968). Eight of the 12 participants experienced at least one episode that was a journey, OBE, or a visitation; the data suggests that they achieved an altered state of consciousness. There were a total of 13 such episodes for the 35 individual sessions.

This research seems to support the theories that suggest that the use of percussion by indigenous cultures in ritual and ceremony has specific neurophysiological effects and is associated with temporary changes in brainwave activity, which may facilitate imagery and entry into an altered state of consciousness. The tempo of each drumbeat used in this study, as it relates to beats per second, appears to be correlated with resulting temporary changes in EEG band power, provided the drumming pattern is sustained for at least 13–15 minutes.

The change is most prominent at minute 9, most notably for theta and alpha waves. According to field observations and subjective reports, the period of time required for most individuals to be affected/inducted by ritual drumming appears to be 13 to 15 minutes (Cade & Coxhead, 1979; Achterberg, 1981; Benson, 1980, 1984; Murphy & Donovan, 1988). This observation echoes the oral teachings of some indigenous cultures concerning auditory stimulation (Arrien, 1989).

Our data showed a rapid increase or diminishment of theta and/or alpha to the 15-minute point, with a gradual gain or diminishment on to the 20-minute point (Figures 2.1, 2.2, 2.3). The drumming pattern most often associated with increased theta wave activity was 4 to 4 1/2 beats per second, or the typical drumming tempo observed in shamanic work. Seven of the 12 participants showed varying degrees of increased theta during the shamanic drumming (Figures 2.2 and 2.5).

Finally, subjects "set and setting" are important, and any replication attempts should keep this in mind. By closing the subjects in a sound-proofed, light-proofed chamber, in a comfortable lying position with their eyes closed, there was an attempt to replicate the postures and conditions typical of the indigenous ceremonies at issue. It seems likely that both the indigenous environment and that in the lab helped participants focus their attention as completely as possible on the auditory stimulation. It also seems intuitive that driving is dependent on the attentional state of a subject: that wandering attention would prevent driving from taking effect, though this cannot be determined from our study. The length of the sessions, almost an hour in total, including baselines before and after the period of stimulation, may also have contributed to the relaxation and attentional processes of the participants. In sum, these factors were likely significant in the successful replication of ritual conditions: not only was an EEG driving response recorded, with concomitant elevations in alpha and theta band power, but the subjective data indicated that participants did indeed undergo a change in state of consciousness.

PART II. EFFECTS OF RHYTHMIC CHANTING ON HEART RATE AND RESPIRATION

Physiological rhythms are hierarchically organized. One rhythm we can (at least partially) control is breathing. However, due to the hierarchical organization of respiratory system, conscious control of breathing influences other physiological rhythms. For example, breathing influences the most prominent component of heart rate variability, Respiratory Sinus Arrhythmia (RSA) (Heart Rate Variability, 1996; Ray et al., 1999; Jovanov, 2005). Rhythmic breathing has prolonged effects on RSA and generates resonance-like effects on heart rate variability (Lehrer et al., 1999; Vaschillo et al., 2002). Very slow yogic breathing has a similar effect (Jovanov, 2005). A typical example of heart rate variability before and after a slow breathing exercise is presented in Figure 2.7. It can be seen that before the breathing exercise the subject exhibits bursts of very regular RSA; for example, regular sine-wave-like bursts of RSA at time 50 sec and 120 sec. During this time, heart rate variability perfectly follows instantaneous lung volume. After the breathing exercise (at time 1050 sec), the subject exhibits a very regular RSA pattern as seen in the lower plot. However, it can be seen that even during the preparation period the RSA pattern becomes very regular as a result of years of exercise and conditioning.

Rhythmic chanting can be seen as a devotional practice that synchronizes the hierarchy of a subject's bodily rhythms and strengthens the coupling between them. Therefore, during this practice we can expect to see an increased interaction of breathing and heart rate variability, or a larger amplitude of the RSA. An example can be seen in Figure 2.8. The upper plot represents heart rate variability at the beginning of chanting, whereas

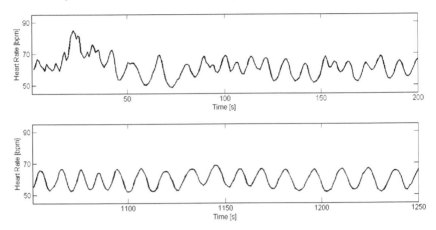

Figure 2.7   The effect of very slow yogic breathing (1 breath/min); heart rate before (upper) and after (lower) this slow breathing exercise (Jovanov, 2005). Heart rate in beats/minute is represented as a function of time in seconds.

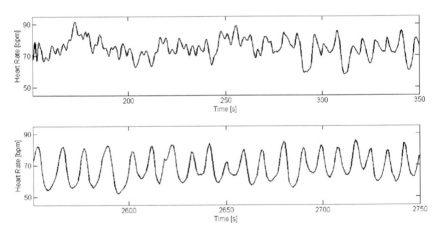

Figure 2.8   The effect of rhythmic chanting, at the beginning of trial (upper plot) and 45 minutes later (lower plot). Both plots represent heart rate in beats/minute as a function of time in seconds.

the lower plot represents the variability of the same subject after 45 minutes of chanting. A rhythmic, regular pattern of inter-beat variability can be clearly seen on the lower plot.

We believe that the stabilization of basic physiological rhythms may serve as a foundation for higher states of consciousness (Jovanov, 1995; Rakovic et al., 1999). The role of the limbic system is crucial for survival, since it makes possible the high priority body activation necessary during times of crisis. However, during these times, this activation influences certain mental content in our flow of thoughts. This results not only in a change in our conscious state, but in the processing of conscious material. As we cannot consciously and directly control the functions of our limbic system, we cannot directly control our stream of consciousness.

We hypothesize that externally stabilized physiological rhythms can result in periods of uninterrupted conscious experience via the indirect stabilization of the limbic system via practices like chanting or controlled breathing. This stabilization (described experientially as "stillness" by many meditators) can allow deep insights and a variety of integrated experiences to emerge (Iyengar, 1993). To paraphrase a frequently used metaphor: You can hardly see deep into the water when there are tumultuous waves on the surface; however, when the water becomes still, you can see all the way to the bottom.

DISCUSSION AND CONCLUSIONS

To understand more about the relationship between these stimulation techniques and their reported effects, much more clinical research is needed, using the combined efforts of scientists, psychologists, ethnomusicologists, and anthropologists. Naive participants, some having had prior preparation, as well as subjects who are familiar with and have been trained for various types of ASCs, should be tested. Brain electrical activity and autonomous nervous system activity should be monitored. Natives who are indigenous to a culture which still holds to and honors the traditional aspects of drumming as an integral part of ritual and ceremony should be tested in a laboratory using recordings of the actual ceremonial drumming of their culture. These results could then be compared to the results of naive and non-naive subjects. Research involving live drumming should be carried out and then compared to taped drumming.[3] It would also be interesting to simultaneously monitor subjects and drummer(s) to observe common patterns and synchronicity of changes. As the technology becomes available, the use of mobile EEG could prove to be crucial to the study of these ritual techniques in context. We hypothesize that the entrainment techniques such as rhythmic drumming, stabilize and regulate basic body rhythms, which has therapeutic value in itself (see Connie Tomaino's comments in Chapter 6), and allow transcendent experiences to emerge. We hypothesize that these entrainment techniques provide extended control of the limbic system, offering one the chance to reduce emotional noise and settle the mind.

ACKNOWLEDGMENTS

The authors are grateful to Gabe Turow for his enthusiasm and help in the preparation of this paper and Udo Will for careful reading and excellent suggestions.

NOTES

1. In the fall of 1986, as a graduate student in a course on core shamanism, Dr. Maxfield experienced her first "drum journey." Unaided by drugs, she experienced vivid visual and somatic imagery, incorporating classic shamanic and archetypal themes. She was surprised and intrigued. She hypothesized that she was entering into an altered state of consciousness of some kind, related to, but not the same as, a meditative state. If this were so, then, she hypothesized, the nature of this experience could be better understood by measuring the electrical activity of the brain with an electroencephalogram machine (EEG) during such a ritual. Three years later, she began her research to determine whether various drumming patterns would be associated with different brainwave activity, as measured by cortical EEG, and to determine if the subjective experience of percussion in general, and rhythmic drumming in particular, would elicit images or sensations with a common theme.

2. In research on imagery, meditation, and relaxation techniques with inexperienced practitioners, it is a common observation that maximal optimal physiological response occurs within the first 10 to 15 minutes of stimulation, after 25 minutes a diminishing return transpires (Benson, 1984; Cade & Coxhead, 1979; Murphy & Donovan, 1988).

3. The experience of listening to drumming through headphones or small speakers is vastly different from feeling the vibrations of a live drum played in front of you. Monitoring the rhythmic bass vibration/tactile elements of drumming could be a critical addition to future experiments on entrainment to percussion.

REFERENCES

Achterberg, J. (1985). *Imagery in healing: Shamanism and modern medicine.* Boston: Shambala.
Arrien, A. (1989). Personal communication.
Banquet, J. P. (1973). Spectral analysis of the EEG in meditation. *Electroencephalography and Clinical Neurophysiology, 35,* 143–151.
Benson, H. (1975). *The relaxation response.* New York: Morrow.
Benson, H. (1984). *Beyond the relaxation response.* New York: Berkley Books.
Cade, G. M., & Coxhead, F. (1979). *The awakened mind, biofeedback and the development of higher states of awareness.* New York: Delacorte Press.
Crawley, A. E. (1912). Drums and cymbals. *Encyclopaedia of Religious Ethics, V,* 89–94.
Drury, N. (1982). *The shaman and the magician.* London: Routledge and Kegan Paul.
Drury, N. (1989). *Elements of shamanism.* Longmead, Shaftesbury, Dorset: Element Books.
Dyro, F. M. (1989). *The EEG handbook.* Boston: Little, Brown and Co.
Eliade, M. (1964). *Shamanism: Archaic techniques of ecstasy.* (W. R. Trask, Trans.). Princeton, NJ: Princeton University Press.
Green, E., & Green, A. (1977). *Beyond biofeedback.* New York: Delta.
Green, E., & Green, A. (1986). Biofeedback and states of consciousness. In B. Wolman & M. Ulman (Eds.), *Handbook of states of consciousness* (pp. 553–589). New York: Van Nostrand Reinhold Co. Ltd.
Guyton, A. C., & Hall, J. E. (2006). *Textbook of medical physiology.* Philadelphia, PA: Elsevier.

Harner, M. J. (1990). *The way of the shaman: A guide to power and healing.* San Francisco: Harper and Row.

Hart, M. (1990). *Drumming at the edge of magic.* New York: Harper Collins.

Heart rate variability. (1996). *European Heart Journal, 17,* 354–381.

I Ching, Book of changes. (3rd ed.). (1950). (R. W. Wilhelm, Trans.; rendered into English by C. F. Baynes). Princeton, NJ: Princeton University Press. (Bollingen Series XIX).

Iyengar, B. K. S. (1993). *Light on the yoga sutras of Patanjali.* San Francisco, CA: Thorsons.

Jilek, W. G. (1974). *Salish Indian mental health and culture change: Psychohygienic and therapeutic aspects of the guardian spirit ceremonial.* Toronto and Montreal: Holt, Rinehart and Winston.

Jovanov, E. (1995). On methodology of EEG analysis during altered states of consciousness. In D. Rakovic & D. Koruga (Eds.), *Consciousness: Challenge of the 21st century science and technology.* Belgrade, Yugoslavia: ECPD, 218–234.

Jovanov, E. (2005). On spectral analysis of heart rate variability during very slow yogic breathing. *Proceedings of the 27th Annual International Conference of the IEEE Engineering in Medicine and Biology Society.* Shanghai, China, 2467–2470.

Lehrer, P., Sasaki, Y., & Saito, Y. (1999). Zazen and cardiac variability. *Psychosomatic Medicine, 61*(6), 812–821.

Ludwig, A. G. (1968). Altered states of consciousness. In R. Prince (Ed.), *Trance and possession states* (pp. 69–95). Montreal: R. M. Bucke Memorial Society, McGill University. Also in C. Tart (Ed.), (1972). *Altered states of consciousness.* (2nd ed.), (pp. 11–24). New York: Anchor/Doubleday.

Murphy, M., & Donovan, S. (1988). *The physical and psychological effects of meditation: A review of contemporary meditation research with a comprehensive bibliography 1931–1988.* San Rafael: Esalen Institute, Study of Exceptional Functioning.

Needham, R. (1979). Percussion and transition. In W. A. Lessa & E. Z. Vogt (Eds.), *Reader in comparative religion* (pp. 311–317). New York: Harper and Row. (Reprinted from Man. 2 [1967], 606–614.)

Neher, A. (1961). Auditory driving observed with scalp electrodes in normal subjects. *EEG and Clinical Neurophysiology, 13,* 449–451.

Prince, R. (1968a). Can the EEG be used in the study of possession states? In R. Prince (Ed.), *Trance and possession states* (pp. 121–137). Montreal: R. M. Bucke Memorial Society, McGill University.

Prince, R. (1968b). Trance and possession states. *Proceedings of the Second Annual Conference of the R. M. Bucke Memorial Society.* Montreal: R. M. Bucke Memorial Society, McGill University, 121–137.

Rakovic, D., Tomasevic, M. Jovanov, E., Radivojevic, V., Sukovic, P., Martinovic, Z., Car, M., . . . Skaric, L., (1999). Electroencephalographic (EEG) correlates of some activities which may alter consciousness: The transcendental meditation technique, musicogenic states, microwave resonance relaxation, healer/healee interaction, and alertness/drowsiness. *Informatica, 23*(3), 399–412.

Ray, G. C., Kaplan, A. Y., & Jovanov, E. (1999). Homeostatic change in the genesis of ECG during yogic breathing. *Journal of the Institution of Engineers* (India), *79*(1), 28–33.

Rouget, G. (1985). *Music and trance: A theory of the relations between music and possession* (B. Beibuyck, Trans.). Chicago: University of Chicago Press.

Spehlmann, R. (1981). *EEG primer.* Amsterdam, New York, Oxford: Elsevier Biomedical Press.

Tart, C. T. (Ed.). (1972). *Altered states of consciousness* (2nd ed.). Garden City, NY: Anchor Books, Doubleday and Co., Inc.

Vaschillo, E., Lehrer, P., Rishe, N., & Konstantinov, M. (2002). Heart rate variability biofeedback as a method for assessing baroreflex function: A preliminary study of resonance in the cardiovascular system. *Applied Psychophysiology Biofeedback, 27*(1), 1–27.

Wallace, R. K., & Benson, H. (1972). The physiology of meditation. *Scientific American, 226*, 84.

Walsh, R. (1989). Shamanism and early human technology: The technology of transcendence. *Revision, 12*(1), 34–40.

Walsh, R. (1990). *The spirit of shamanism*. Los Angeles: Jeremy P. Tarcher.

3 Rhythmic Entrainment and Evolution

Judith Becker

INTRODUCTION

Moving in synchrony with members of one's community, and in synchrony with music played specifically for one's community, often results in feelings of bondedness with the co-participants. The emotional rush a person may feel in such situations may go far beyond communal goodwill, reaching up to and including transcendent feelings of union with a holy power, or the rapturous feeling of the loss of a personal I. Sometimes, the music itself seems to subsume all single identities and the lock-step swaying or dancing is experienced as being one with the music. Roland Barthes (1986) writes of the body in a state of music and it is T. S. Eliot (1943) who says, you are the music while the music lasts.

The strongest case for the power of rhythmic music to elicit deep emotional responses occurs in situations of group response, of near-unison swaying that occurs spontaneously. Examples include a Pentecostal religious service or a rock concert (Sylvan, 2005). From the observer's viewpoint, the group acts almost as a single organism, while the participant feels a unity with all other members present, a oneness that at least temporarily overrides differences of class, gender, ethnicity, or personal politics. While isolated, individual musical listening undoubtedly can stimulate feelings of rapture, but the group experience trumps all for sheer ecstatic musical listening.

Group rhythmic entrainment is a prime catalyst for musical ecstasy. Why should this be so? The term rhythmic entrainment is sometimes used in two different senses, depending upon one's disciplinary allegiances. As discussed in Chapter 1, the scientific community distinguishes between synchrony, moving in unison, and rhythmic entrainment, which requires that:

- There be two or more autonomous rhythmic processes or oscillators, and
- The oscillators interact (Clayton, Sager, & Will, 2005).

It has been pointed out that there are innumerable endogenous rhythmic processes or oscillators within a human body (Large, 2001; Janata &

Grafton, 2003); isolating those oscillators that may entrain to rhythmic music is a task of daunting complexity.

Humanists use the term rhythmic entrainment to describe synchronous movements of human bodies in situations of one-on-one human interaction starting at birth (Condon, 1986), in intercultural group situations involving language such as classrooms (Erickson & Mohatt, 1982), and most particularly musical situations involving groups of people moving in harmony. I am not willing to substitute the term *synchronous behavior* for *rhythmic entrainment* for the kind of work I do. Synchrony doesn't capture the power of the interaction. Synchrony needs no agency. It might happen accidentally without any conscious intent. Rhythmic entrainment, on the other hand, implies something of the force that the music has upon the listeners and suggests something of the intentions of the music-makers. In groups of people listening to music they love, the extraordinary strength of bodily, intellectual, and affective responses is simply not captured by the term synchrony.

The scientific study of group rhythmic entrainment in the humanistic sense is enormously complicated by the fact that at least four variables are involved:

1. The music;
2. The listening person;
3. The other listening persons; and
4. The environment, the situation, or the context of the musical listening.

Given the fact that scientific studies cannot proceed with so many variables of such internal complexity, nearly all psychological and neurological studies of rhythmic entrainment deal only with two variables: the music itself, and the listening individual, and ignore context entirely.

Much of the work on entrainment by neuroscientists thus necessarily focuses on entrainment within a single body. Studying endogenous rhythmic entrainment as well as cross-body entrainment demands complex technology and special training not normally accessible to those, like myself, in humanistic disciplines. From the early studies of music and the brain such as Neher's early work in the 1960s (Neher, 1961) analyzing the brain rhythms of subjects listening to drum beats in a laboratory, to the more recent works of Clynes (1986), Maxfield (1990), Wallin (1991), Clayton et al. (2005), and many others, musical scholars have adopted the scientific model and studied single brains in isolation.

Studies in music cognition have largely followed the empirical models of cognitive studies in general in their efforts to model the algorithms of single brains processing music (Raffman, 1993; Lerdahl & Jackendoff, 1983). Neurophysiologists and psychologists of consciousness likewise follow the dictates of their scientific training, isolating and narrowing the problem as much as possible in order to have some control over the variables. The development of technologies such as magnetic resonance imaging (fMRI) and positron emission tomography (PET) scanning have reinforced the practice of the study of single minds in the attempt to unravel the power and mysteries of musical experience (Blood & Zatorre, 2001; Janata, Tillman, & Bharucha, 2002; Menon & Levitin, 2005). In spite of the inherent limitations of single-brain studies, it still may be possible to extrapolate results from single-brain musical studies in order to hypothesize what is happening in a group musical situation.

RESEARCH ON DEEP LISTENERS

The results of a recent study by the author and her research assistant, Joshua Penman, on musical listening and emotion support the assumption that what happens in the laboratory may be seen as a somewhat diminished reflection of what happens in a group situation. The focus of the study was not rhythmic entrainment, but rather to test the hypothesis put forward in my book, *Deep Listeners: Music, Emotion and Trancing* (2004). The hypothesis was that religious ecstatics and those I call *deep listeners* (those persons who have profoundly emotional reactions to musical listening), exhibit Galvanic Skin Response[1] (GSR) profiles more like each other than like control groups. In other words, we hypothesized that deep listeners have a stronger emotional/physiological response to music than non-deep listeners, which may begin to explain why some people spontaneously enter religious trance when their peers do not. Demonstrating that there was a statistical difference between groups in GSR response was an attempt to use a data-driven method to confirm that deep listeners have a different physiology than non-deep listeners.

As a follow-up to the single-person GSR testing in my office, a few of the Pentecostal ecstatics were tested in church during a worship service. The comparative GSR readings and heart rate readings demonstrated increased emotional arousal in the group church context as compared with the office setting. Although the participants were asked to sit quietly during the service so as not to disturb the heart rate and GSR graphs, their co-worshippers were almost all moving in time with the music. What follows is a description of the Pentecostal ecstatics and deep listeners study and some of the conclusions.

DESCRIPTION OF STUDY[2]

Participants

In this experiment, the participants (n = 60) were divided into five groups; two were target groups, those we wished to compare with all others.

The target groups were the Pentecostal Ecstatics and the Deep Listeners. These were the two populations that were hypothesized as having stronger emotional reactions to music they love than do other groups. The comparison groups were Pentecostal Non-Ecstatics; members of two other Protestant churches, designated as Other Protestants, and participants recruited from the general student population of the author's university, called General Students. Thus, the two target groups, Pentecostal Ecstatics and Deep Listeners, were not randomly selected (nor could they be). The Pentecostal Ecstatics were separated out from the Pentecostals in general, and the Deep Listeners were self-selected as persons profoundly moved by listening to music. The Pentecostal Ecstatics and the Pentecostal Non-Ecstatics were drawn from a local Apostolic Faith Pentecostal church. The church is multi-racial with a middle-to-lower-middle-class demographic and about 500 members. The congregation was told that the authors were conducting a study on music and emotion.

The classification *ecstatic* was made solely on the basis of observation: if, during one of the many church services the authors attended, participants were seen to trance, they were classified as ecstatics. Within the church, the particular manifestations of trance are speaking in tongues, translating of the speaking in tongues by someone else who is also in trance, shaking and trembling with upraised arms, anguished facial expressions, and often the classic collapse onto the ground that signals the end of trance (Rouget, 1985). These trance manifestations are often combined, as for example, shaking and trembling with an anguished facial expression, or, speaking in tongues, trembling with upraised arms, followed by the collapse onto the floor. Whereas the possibility exists that the trancing of one or more of the participants was missed, generally speaking, those who trance at all do so on a fairly regular basis.

Members of two other local churches were recruited as one of the comparison groups (Other Protestants). These churches (Vineyard Christian Fellowship and Crossroads Community Baptist) are similar to the Pentecostal church in demographics (working-class and multi-racial, though predominantly white) and in their worship music (Christian Rock and soft Gospel). There is, however, no trance component to their services. This group included some people whose GSR graphs indicated strong responses to musical listening, and thus people who, according to my hypothesis, are potential trancers were ecstatic practices condoned or encouraged in their churches.

The Deep Listeners were recruited from friends and colleagues of the authors at the school of music of their university. An e-mail message was sent to all faculty members of the school of music, and several music school classes were visited to describe the study. In both cases, the authors asked for volunteers who believed themselves to be deep listeners. They were mainly music students and professors.

In response to the query on the questionnaire,

Do you think that your responses (to music) are:
- the same as
- less strong than
- stronger than
. . . those of your friends?

nearly all subjects checked "stronger than"—hardly surprising for people who have devoted their lives to music. The General Student group was recruited by means of signs posted in public places around the university. The participants who responded were all students pursuing undergraduate degrees.

The groups do not, therefore, have the same criteria for inclusion. The Pentecostal Ecstatics and Pentecostal Non-Ecstatics were designated by the authors based upon observed behavior at church. The Deep Listeners were self-selected based upon their declared emotional response to musical listening, whereas the Other Protestants and General Students groups were randomly selected.

To rule out the cultural suspicion that trancers may not be mentally stable, a psychiatric exam was performed on 9 Pentecostal Ecstatics and 10 Pentecostal Non-Ecstatics with the Hamilton Depression Inventory, the Brief Psychiatric Rating Scale, the Mini Mental State Examination, and the Schedule for the Assessment of Negative Symptoms (SANS). These findings affirmed that the ecstatics exhibited no psychological symptoms that indicated that the ecstatic states that were observed and identified as trance could have been due to psychopathological conditions. Whereas a few individuals were identified who had affective symptoms such as depression or hypomania, in no case were any found who would meet clinical criteria for depersonalization, fugue, psychosis, multiple personality, or associated disorders. The only outwardly discernable difference between the Pentecostal Ecstatic category and the Pentecostal Non-Ecstatic category is that the ecstatics are likely to trance during religious services whereas the non-ecstatics do not.

Materials

The participants' GSR was measured using Ag-AgCl2 electrodes attached to the index finger and the middle finger (Stern, Ray, & Quigley, 2001). Heart Rate was measured using a pulse photoplethysmogram transducer attached to the thumb. All were connected to a BIOPAC MP100 system, and recorded on a Macintosh computer using the AcqKnowledge software program.

Procedures

All participants were asked to bring in two favorite songs or pieces of music. The advantages of participant-selected versus experimenter-selected music often outweightthemoreuniformapproachofusingonlyexperimenter-selectedmusic (e.g., Harrer & Harrer, 1977; Thaut & Davis, 1993; Rickard, 2004). The aim of this study was to compare GSR of different groups while listening to music that was cherished by each participant. Thus, both participant-selected music and experimenter-selected music (as a control) were called for. After completing the questionnaire and the consent form, the participant was given headphones and sat on a comfortable couch looking out a window with a pleasant view. This spatial arrangement was intended to minimize the effect of having the experimenters and the equipment in the same room as the participant.

After an initial quiet period of 2–3 minutes, the following musical excerpts were played, allowing a 1-minute period of silence between each excerpt:

1. Control 1: 3rd movement from Symphony in F major, J-C 38, by Giovanni Battista Sammartini
2. Participant Selection 1: First of the participant's favorite pieces
3. Control 2: Favorite music of another participant
4. Participant Selection 2: Second of the participant's favorite pieces

For the first control, a work by the minor early-Classical composer Sammartini was chosen. The rationale for this choice is that, according to our evaluation, the work was of such inoffensive blandness that no one would respond strongly to it. (As it turned out, many of the Deep Listeners, in fact, did.)

The second control example was chosen from a small number of pieces that had been the favorite music of earlier participants. These included "Bad Habits," by Destiny's Child, "A Thousand Years," by Sting, and "Tricycle Built for Two," by Mr. Laurence. These were all pieces that had engendered intense reactions in the participants who initially brought them in. The rationale for this was to suggest that the physiological response to music is not inherent in the music itself, but rather resides in the relationship between a specific listener and that music. It is generally assumed that one's emotional reaction is exclusively related to features intrinsic to the music itself. Among ethnomusicologists, and among those musicologists who have worked on this issue (Meyer, 1956), it is clear that one's response to musical stimuli is a complex of emotional reactions relating to familiarity, to texts, to previous musical associations, to previous situational associations, as well as what may be called purely musical considerations. The fact that one of our control examples was an emotional stimulant to one person, and a neutral control for another is to be expected. At the end of the experiment, participants were asked about their experiences with listening to music in general, and with listening to music in the experiment in particular.

GSR Index

We calibrated each recording by setting the baseline to zero. We then removed the system noise using a digital lowpass filter with a cutoff frequency of 2Hz. The GSR was recorded as an AC signal, thereby measuring only changes in conductance. This means that when conductance was steady, the GSR signal was flat at 0. When the participant's GSR changed, the graphical output reflected these changes by peaks and troughs. For ease of calculation, the changes in GSR were measured in units of 1 = .2 μmhos. Because participants' responses to the music were distributed over the whole listening period, we found it most productive to treat the participants GSR recordings for each given example as a unit, calculating the GSR Index, which assigns a single value for the integrated GSR reading. To compute these values, we rectified the AC signal by taking the absolute value of the recording and then integrating the area between the curve and baseline. The GSR Index was then calculated by dividing this integral by the length of the excerpt. The GSR Index, then, is an aggregate measure of the strength of a given participant's response to a piece of music. Contrary to the literature that stresses the habituation effect of musical listening with GSR (e.g., Eisenstein, Eisenstein, & Bonheim, 1991; Aramaki, Kira, & Hirasawa, 1997; Toyokura, 1998; Tarvainenn et al., 2001, p. 1071), we found no general diminution of response across time, either within a particular example, or across successive examples (Figure 3.1).

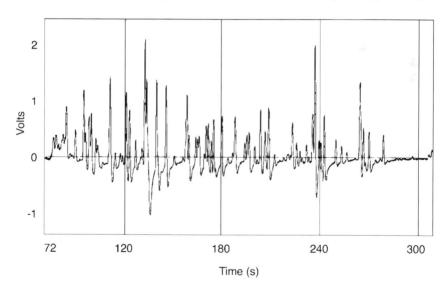

Figure 3.1 The Calibrated and low-pass filtered GSR recording of one participant while listening to one of her self-selected pieces. Notice the lack of habituation that would result in a GSR line with diminishing peaks.

Heart Rate

Heart rate is another standard measure of arousal; both sympathetic and parasympathetic branches of the ANS may be involved in changes in heart rate (e.g., Witvliet & Vrana, 1995; Krumhansl, 1997; Stern et al., 2001; Rickard, 2004). For each excerpt, the mean and standard deviation of the heart rate of the participants were calculated. This was done using the Find Rate function of the AcqKnowledge software program that translates a pulse recording into rate data. It was necessary to discard a fair amount of spurious data due to the susceptibility of pulse photoplethysmogram measurements to errors.

Music

The musical preferences of the participants were quite diverse, and related to the social group to which they belonged.

Table 3.1   The Genres of Music Selected by Each Participant Group

	Pentecostal Ecstatics	Deep Listeners	Pentecostal Non-Ecstatics	Other Protestants	General Students
n	*20*	*28*	*32*	*16*	*24*
Contemporary Christian	30% *(6)*		63% *(20)*	50% *(8)*	
Classical		57% *(16)*	3% *(1)*	13% *(2)*	
Pop					17% *(4)*
Rock/Alternative	15% *(3)*	18% *(5)*	16% *(5)*	6% *(1)*	50% *(12)*
Rap/R&B			3% *(1)*		13% *(3)*
Gospel	40% *(8)*		16% *(5)*	13% *(2)*	
Electronic					13% *(3)*
New Age				13% *(2)*	8% *(2)*
World	10% *(2)*	18% *(5)*			
Children's				6% *(1)*	
Jazz	5% *(1)*	7% *(2)*			

All three church groups, Pentecostal Ecstatics, Pentecostal Non-Ecstatics, and Other Protestants included a substantial percentage of religious music in their selections. Only the Deep Listeners category included a substantial percentage of classical music, whereas Rock/Alternative music was selected by a substantial percentage of the General Students category.

RESULTS

GSR Index

The GSR Index for the two participant-selected pieces and the GSR Index for the two control pieces were averaged for each participant. The assumption was that the participant would display a similar profile to both of his/her selected pieces and likewise, a similar profile to both of the control pieces. This turned out to be the case: There was not a statistically significant difference by a paired-samples t-test between the GSR Index for the two participant-selected pieces (p = .658), nor for the two control pieces (p = .330). Based upon the GSR Index for participant-selected music, 2 participants were discarded as outliers, as their values were more than 3 standard deviations above the mean. One outlier was in the General Students group with an GSR Index of 31.8, and the other was in the Other Protestants group with an GSR Index of 29.0. The graphs for GSR Index for participant-selected

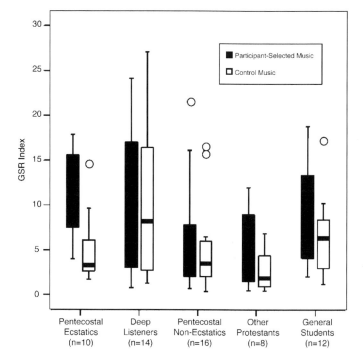

Figure 3.2 GSR Index compared across groups. Statistical analysis of GSR index values across groups. For each individual we computed separate GSR index values for their own selections and the control selections. The dark horizontal line represents the median value for the group, the boxes represent the values for the middle 50 percent of subjects, and the whiskers represent the full range of responses except for the circles which represent single subjects. This graphical convention will be used throughout the article.

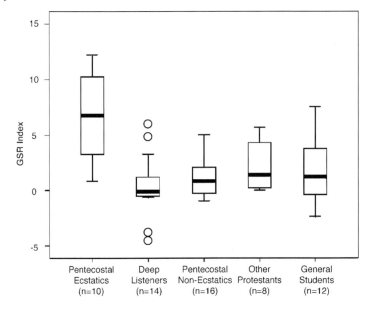

Figure 3.3   Difference of GSR Index compared across groups. GSR Index for participant-selected music minus GSR Index for control music, indicating the strong preference for participant-selected music by the Pentecostal Ecstatics.

musics that indicate the highest readings were in the Pentecostal Ecstatics group and the Deep Listeners group. The graphs for Deep Listeners for the control music is higher than that for all groups, and is, in fact, little different from their self-selected music (statistical significance was revealed by a one-way ANOVA completed for the GSR Index for participant-selected music across the groups (F [1, 61] = 2.83, p = 0.033). The following comparative differences between groups in GSR Index for participant-selected music are statistically significant by LSD: Pentecostal Ecstatics versus Other Protestants (p = 0.018); Pentecostal Ecstatics versus Pentecostal Non-Ecstatics (p = 0.018); Deep Listeners versus Pentecostal Non-Ecstatics (p = .025); and Deep Listeners versus Other Protestants (p = 0.026).

In this study, the difference between the GSR of the Pentecostal Ecstatics to their music (mostly religious) and the control music was far greater than that difference in all the other groups. This measurement also highlights the fact that many in the Deep Listeners category unexpectedly responded strongly to the control example, resulting in a minimal difference of the responses between their self-selected music and the control music. It may be very difficult to find any music that those in the Deep Listeners group would not respond to. None of the groups was homogenous, in terms of their GSR, to music they chose. In every group there were persons who responded strongly and persons who responded weakly in terms of GSR while listening to music they loved. Within this diversity, however, certain profiles appeared.

Heart Rate

The differences in mean heart rate between participant-selected and control music were calculated. This is the only way that heart rate data can
be used, since everyone comes to the experiment with a different baseline
heart rate. Because of problems recording the pulse of some participants,
the heart rate data comes from only 55 participants. Four of the participants whose data is unused are in the General Students group; 1 is in the
Pentecostal Ecstatics group. There was a statistically significant (mean
difference = 2.10, p = 0.002) difference in participants' responses to each
of their self-selected pieces. That is, participants had a lower average heart
rate for their second selection. Nevertheless, we are choosing to average these two heart rates for ease of comparison. The average difference
between the heart rates for the control pieces, however, was not significant (p = .691). In the literature, musical listening and heart rate measurements have revealed widely differing profiles. Sometimes heart rate
increases and sometimes decreases with musical listening (e.g., Hodges,
1980; Davis & Thaut, 1989). In this study, all of the groups demonstrated
a greater mean heart rate while listening to self-selected musical examples
compared to control examples.

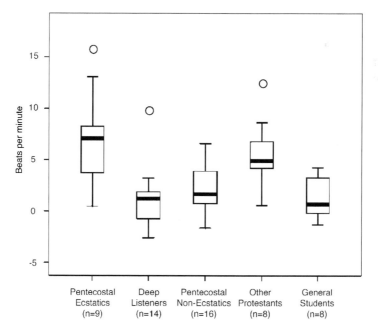

Figure 3.4 Difference of average heart rate. The difference across
groups between average heart rate for participant-selected pieces and
average heart rate for control pieces.

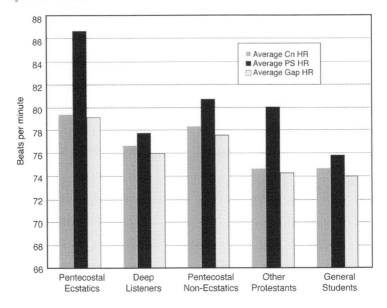

Figure 3.5 Average HR for participant-selected piece compared with control and no-music. Chart demonstrating the increase in heart rate across groups when listening to their own music compared with the control music or the no music situation (Cn = control music, PS = participant-selected music).

SUPPLEMENTAL FINDINGS

In the course of this study, a number of findings emerged that, whereas they were not the focus of the guiding hypotheses, they provoked their own interest and also relate to previous studies of the physiological aspects of music and emotion. One of these observations concerned the Intensity Level of the participant-selected listening examples.

Intensity Level (IL)

The correlation, or not, between powerful music and strength of emotional response has been tested before (e.g., Zimny & Weidenfeller, 1963; Thaut, 1990; Rickard, 2004), with results generally indicating stronger response to powerful music than to more calm music. In order to determine if GSR Index was correlated with features such as tempo, loudness, register, and timbre that could be construed as increasing powerfulness, the authors devised the measurement Intensity Level (IL). IL is a subjective measurement of how intense each piece of music was. Both authors have extensive musical backgrounds and thus felt qualified to make such an evaluation. IL

Table 3.2 Mean Intensity Level (IL) for Each of the Five Groups of Participants

Mean Intensity Level (IL) for each of the five groups of participants

	Mean IL
Pentecostal Ecstatics	5.35
Deep Listeners	5.31
Pentecostal Non-Ecstatics	5.48
Other Protestants	4.06
General Students	5.33

is a subjective rating that combines tempo, loudness, register, and timbre. For each selection, the authors independently came up with an intensity rating on a 9-point scale. The ratings arrived at by the authors were usually the same, and only twice did they differ by more than one point.

These subjective ratings were averaged to calculate the Intensity Level (IL) score for each piece. Most musical examples were in the mid-range, with a few at either end of the continuum.

Listed below are typical examples of the ratings:

Level

1. Level 1: "Only Time," by Enya
2. Level 2: "When I Fall in Love," by Chris Botti
3. Level 3: "I Wont Last a Day without You," by David Osborne
4. Level 4: "Michele," by The Beatles
5. Level 5: "Water Night," by Eric Whitacre
6. Level 6: "On the Nickel," by Tom Waits
7. Level 7: "Stigmatized," by The Calling
8. Level 8: "Bold as Love," by Jimi Hendrix
9. Level 9: "I'm Going Through," by Aretha Franklin

It was found that GSR Index is moderately correlated to Intensity Level for the participant-selected music. For the first participant-selected piece, the Spearman correlation coefficient between GSR Index and IL is 0.38 (p = .0042); for the second piece, it is 0.26 (p = .048).

Differences Between GSR Peaks in Office and in Church

Nearly all the Pentecostal participants volunteered the information that they experienced stronger arousal in church than in my office, thus supporting the assertion made earlier that group musical experience is often

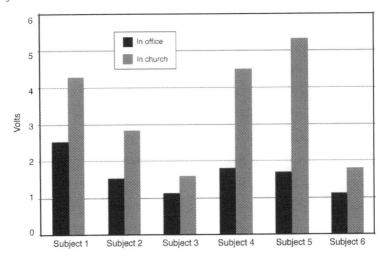

Figure 3.6   Comparison between GSR peaks of six Pentecostal ecstatics in office test situation and in church service showing greater arousal in group musical context.

more intense than single-person listening. To support this hypothesis, we measured the GSR peaks of a few of the Pentecostal Ecstatics during an actual church service. We then compared the strongest response to a musical example during the church service with the strongest response that same individual exhibited while listening to their favorite music in the office. The results were entirely predictable and reinforce the idea that, at some point, context needs to be considered within scientific studies of rhythmic entrainment and musical emotions.

DISCUSSION

The initial hypotheses of this study predicted that the Pentecostal Ecstatics and Deep Listeners would have a stronger GSR Index to listening to music they love than other groups. With respect to GSR Index for participant-selected music, the Pentecostal Ecstatics and the Deep Listeners, in fact, demonstrated stronger responses than all other groups, and with statistically significant results, compared with the Pentecostal Non-Ecstatics and Other Protestant groups. Another similarity between ecstatics and deep listeners, not pursued here, is that both often describe their listening experiences in transcendent terms. For example, ecstatics and deep listeners, in interviews connected with this study and in the literature on strong emotions and musical listening, speak of the loss of boundaries between self and other, or experiences of wholeness and unity, or of a nearness to the sacred (e.g.,

Gabrielsson & Lindstrom, 1993; Gabrielsson & Wik, 2000; Gabrielsson, 2001; Becker, 2004). The General Students scored lower in terms of GSR Index than both the Pentecostal Ecstatics and Deep Listeners, but those differences are not statistically significant.

It is possible that when deep listeners are put in a church setting at a young age that they learn to amplify and exaggerate their response to music until it achieves ecstatic proportions. In that way, they are actually learning to be deeper listeners: They have a biological predisposition to be stimulated by music, but because of their environment and culture, they learn to gradually cultivate that response, making it even more intense and exaggerated over the years. These findings support statements by all our Pentecostal participants that they experience greater arousal in church than in a laboratory setting. Even while sitting quietly, but within the context of group rhythmic entrainment, the Pentecostal ecstatics registered stronger arousal when surrounded by swaying, clapping, and singing co-parishioners.

IMPLICATIONS OF STUDY

Supra-Individual Biological Processes

The commonly acknowledged fact that group rhythmic entrainment contributes to feelings of ecstasy points to the importance of studies in what Rafael Nuñez calls supra-individual biological processes (Nuñez, 1997). Nuñez uses the example of linguistic accents to help one think about this way of approaching human experience. A linguistic accent can be attributable to a particular individual, but it is not the creation of a particular individual—it results from historical processes of language imitation and repetition.

Musical events usually entail a number of individuals participating in fairly prescribed roles. The pastor or ritual practitioner may not be a musician, or a musician may not be an audience member, or neither of them may be a dancer. Everyone knows who are the appropriate musicians, ritual practitioners, and dancers; these boundaries are maintained. Yet, the phenomenon of rhythmic entrainment is transpersonal, does not take place in one particular mind alone, although it also takes place there. The dancing and musicking are ways in which a group of people may be-in-the-world. And by their being-in-the-world they communally bring forth the world in which rhythmic entrainment is a natural, expected, un-sensational occurrence. No one person is responsible, no one person is existentially alone, there is no solitary consciousness observing the world, nor even a unitary self-contained being. The group acts as a unit, including ritual practitioners, patient (if there is one), dancers, musicians, on-lookers, even hecklers in some situations become part of a larger, on-going, largely predictable event. The world brought forth by all the participants makes possible the extraordinary moves of the ritual practitioner, or the endurance of the dancers, or the inspiration of the musicians; what may on another day seem strange, is coherent, reasonable, truthful, and authentic within the situation itself.

Structural Coupling and Rhythmic Entrainment

In spite of the overwhelming single-brain, single-body emphasis found within scientific studies, there are scholars who are working to establish methods for cross-subject brain studies that bear on group rhythmic entrainment. I am using the term *structural coupling* developed by Maturana and Varela (1987) to describe a process that encompasses single cell organisms up to human social groups to help imagine what happens when groups of like-minded people are involved in recurrent situations of shared music. Maturana and Varela's usage extends from interactions of single cells to multicellular organisms, to groups of mammals, to include human communities.

I believe that the biological notion of structural coupling is more helpful than the model of traditional cognitive studies in understanding the phenomenon of rhythmic entrainment and of the emotional effect of musical performance and musical listening. Rhythmic entrainment can be seen as structural coupling, of a changed interior, as a personal consciousness in a musical domain of coordination. Bodies and brains synchronize gestures, muscle actions, breathing (Haas, Distenfeld, & Axen, 1986), and seemingly, brainwaves (Neher, 1961; Zakharova & Avdeev, 1982; Maxfield, 1990; Will & Berg, 2007) while enveloped in music. Many persons, bound together by common aims, may experience revitalization and general good feeling. The situation is communal and individual, music descends upon all alike, whereas each person's joy is his or her own.

Rhythmic entrainment is usually thought of in terms of large groups of people participating in a common activity like dancing, singing, or listening to music. But coordinating bodily rhythms may have a much more fundamental, more primal evolutionary development than we normally assume.

Within the human community, rhythmic entrainment begins within minutes after birth. A new-born baby will demonstrate interactional synchrony with a caregiver within the first half-hour of its life (Benzon, 2001). Using what he calls micro-behavioral analysis William Condon has shown that speakers and listeners become immediately entrained to each other's speech rhythms. The dance of the speaker becomes the dance of the listener. Whatever body parts the listener happens to be moving at that moment will be organized and will follow the organization of the speaker's speech. Further, the listener's body often speeds up and slows down in relation to the softness or loudness of the speaker's speech (Condon, 1986).

Our speech and our body motions exhibit wave-like characteristics that are both personal and cultural. Differences between the speech rhythms and the body rhythms of different cultural subgroups within the U.S. are often the source of profound dis-ease between, say, mid-western Protestants and New York Jews, as has been vividly illustrated by Deborah Tannen (1984). Frederick Erickson has studied the differences between the cultural rhythms of two teachers in classrooms at the Odawa Indian Reserve (Algonquin) in Northern Ontario in Canada; one teacher was an Odawa, the other a white American (Erickson & Mohatt, 1982). Both were skilled, experienced teachers. He made videotapes of their respective classrooms during a lesson and then analyzed the tapes frame by frame to discern the rhythms of the students in relation to their teachers, a technique he calls microethnography. In a lecture-demonstration given at the University of Michigan, Erickson showed a video of the American teacher he studied in which there was clear dis-synchrony in his classroom: a lack of smoothly coordinated actions between the teacher and students. Their rhythms were out-of-sync. Erickson then switched tapes to show the classroom with the Native American teacher; the on-video movements of students and teacher were so well synchronized that Erickson was able to slowly and rhythmically wave his arms with the movements of the teacher and students. According to the study, the teacher whose rhythms were entrained with those of her students had a more successful class, and it seems reasonable to assume that their mutually coordinated rhythms were a contributing factor. If speech rhythms can entrain, how much more powerful is musical entrainment with a pulse that penetrates to our bones, with melodies that thrill, and a cosmology that gives life meaning and purpose?

What is Gained by Claiming these Processes as Biological?

If we think of music-making within a ritual that may also include preaching, glossolalia, and dancing—as part of a biological/historical process that has had a long tradition of continual self-recreation—we can begin to think of the music and every other aspect of the ritual process as contributing to bringing forth the activities of each other: as bringing forth a world, a reality in which certain actions are expected and appropriate, and in which the reality brought forth by all is enacted by all. A music event is not just in the minds of the participants, it is in their bodies; like a language accent, playing and listening to music are personally manifested but exist supra-individually. All persons involved—musicians, preachers, or DJs, and other participants—seem to be acting as self-contained, bounded individuals, and indeed they experience whatever they experience as deeply personal and emotional, but the event as a whole plays itself out in a supra-individual domain. Language, music, and dance become a system of ontogenic coordination of actions. Together, they bring about changes in being, and changes in the ritual involved. Whereas it is the individual who experiences ecstasy, it is the group and its domain of coordination that triggers ecstasy. There must be changes in the neurophysiology of the ecstatic for ecstasy to occur, but those changes are not attributable simply to the brain/body of a self-contained individual. They occur through the group processes of recurrent interactions between co-defined individuals in a rhythmic domain of music that is intrinsically social, visibly embodied, and profoundly cognitive.

We may claim that special modes of conscious experience that emerge in situations that involve rhythmic entrainment and emotional responses to music listening emerge as phenotypic features of humankind, as biological developments in the evolution of the species, emerging from both genetic and environmental influences. Emotion, music, and rhythmic entrainment—viewed as evolving together in the interaction of each individual with performances throughout his/her life—dissolves intractable dichotomies concerning nature verses culture, and scientific universalism versus cultural particularism. Culture can be understood as a supra-individual biological phenomenon, a transgenerational history of ongoing social structural couplings that become embodied in the individual and transmitted through future actions.

Music listeners as well as musicians undergo a learning process in which they imitate physical and mental gestures that ultimately transform both their inner structures as well as their relations to everything beyond the boundaries of their skins. Music and emotion are part of a larger processual event that subsumes many other people doing many other things while the whole event unfolds as a unity that has been organized and re-organized over time by small structural changes within the participants. Groups of people who are focused on a common event and who share a common history of that event, act, react, and to some extent think in concert, without sacrificing their bounded personal identities.

The total event needs to be the unit of analysis, not just the participants, and not just the musicians. Group rhythmic entrainment and music underline the phenomenological necessity of understanding our experiences as including more than our bounded, unitary selves. Whether in the language of Maturana and Varela we speak of structural coupling, or in the language of Nuñez we talk of supra-individual biological processes, or the language of Oughourlian (1991) as interdividual processes, the analysis of rhythmic entrainment and music benefits from thinking about the transformations as not happening solely inside a particular body, but happening across several, or many bodies. This approach is helpful in looking at any musical occurrence, and helps to nudge us away from our cultural/intuitive sense that what happens in musical events happens exclusively within a particular body, rather than across bodies, in which each individual may be playing a different role, but in which the entrainment and musicking are not localized within one individual. The advantages of this approach are that we are discouraged from trying to look inside a particular brain/body to find the answers to the special aura that such events have, but are looking rather at the aura of the whole. The event is not coded in the culture or even in an individual. It is an enactment, a performance by particular groups of persons who continually restructure each other and subsequent events.

Emotions can usefully be viewed as being about an individual within a community, rather than being exclusively about internal states. First-person descriptions of music and emotion are rife with tropes of interiority, yet the understanding of how music affects interiors takes place within consensual, shared views of what makes up reality. Musical events set up an aural domain of coordination that envelops all those present. Rhythmic entrainment, though experienced in a particular body, seems never to be bounded by that single body. Emotion, music, and dance become one system of ontogenic coordination of actions. Together, they bring about changes in being and changes in the music event involved. Whereas it is the individual who experiences the emotion, it is the group and its domain of coordinations that triggers the emotion. The changes in the neurophysiology of the listener are not attributable simply to the brain and body of a self-contained individual. They occur through group processes of recurrent interactions between co-defined individuals in a rhythmic domain of music. Thinking of the relationship of emotion and music and rhythmic entrainment as a biological process with a co-defined, historically enacted ontology—as a group creation in which self-contained individuals have undergone structural changes through their interaction with other self-contained individuals—helps to provide an integrated embodied analysis of the relationship of music and emotion and rhythmic entrainment.

Rhythmic Entrainment and Evolution

If the imbrication of music, emotion, and rhythmic entrainment is envisioned as a continuously evolving process of an individual interacting with other individuals, *then musical/ rhythmic entrainment may be considered as assisting in the evolution of the species.* Synchronizing bodies and actions in musical performance appears to be a unique characteristic of our species (Merker, 2000; Freeman, 2000) and may have evolutionary implications in terms of facilitating group activities directed toward finding food or fighting enemies. Scholars such as William Benzon (2001) and Walter Freeman (2000) have made bold claims concerning the evolutionary importance of musical entrainment. Freeman suggests that musical entrainment has been a powerful tool with clear evolutionary advantages for forging a sense of identification between individuals and within groups of individuals. (Freeman, 2000). He believes that something like musical entrainment has served as a survival necessity given the solipsism of the human brain.

Freeman's use of the word solipsism is referring to the demonstrated biological fact that our perception of the world outside of ourselves does not directly reflect sensory inputs, but is a complex construction involving many areas of the brain in addition to those mainly involved with perception.

Thus, our mental images, our inner representations of the outside world, may overlap with those of others in some ways, but are always in some sense sui generis. Freeman thus sees the necessity for some mechanism to overcome this solipsism and finds it in communal music and dancing. He uses the term trance to refer to the feeling of loss of self, of unity with others that occurs in situations of rhythmic entrainment.

I conclude that music and dance originated through biological evolution of brain chemistry, which interacted with the cultural evolution of behavior. This led to the development of chemical and behavioral technology for inducing altered states of consciousness. The role of trance states was particularly important for breaking down preexisting habits and beliefs. That meltdown appears to be necessary for personality changes leading to the formation of social groups by cooperative action leading to trust. Bonding is not simply a release of a neurochemical in an altered state. It is the social action of dancing and singing together that induces new forms of behavior, owing to the malleability that can come through the altered state. It is reasonable to suppose that musical skills played a major role early in the evolution of human intellect, because they made possible formation of human societies as a prerequisite for the transmission of acquired knowledge across generations (Freeman, 2000).

Taking up this theme, Benzon has elaborated and expanded upon the idea of the singular importance of music-making and rhythmic coordination of bodies in the ongoing societal need to overcome private, non-sharable inner lives, and to join in a community of our fellow creatures to build social coherence (Benzon, 2001). Like Freeman, Benzon suggests that the evolution of music and the evolution of man as a social being are coterminous, that communal musical activity and rhythmic entrainment may have facilitated the survival of humankind by facilitating social bonding. Groups working together in hunting, in searching for food, in building shelters, in making clothing, and in raising children have a much better chance of survival than do individuals or single couples. *Musical cohesion becomes a model for social cohesion.* This is an attractive explanation for musical activity that otherwise might seem somewhat peripheral to more goal-oriented activities of humankind—an explanation that overcomes the current tendency to place musical activity outside the mainstream of productive behaviors. Benzon has proposed a basic social principle reliant upon shared musical activity, upon rhythmic entrainment.

The Social Principle: human beings create a uniquely human social space when their nervous systems are coupled through interactional synchrony. (Benzon, 2001)

Benzon uses the term coupling in the same way that Marturana and Varela use structural coupling to mean the mutual biological linkage of one person and another through interaction that affects the structure of both parties.

If the whole village is listening and dancing, then the whole village is enacting a single pattern of musical activity, even though they are physically distinct individuals with distinct nervous systems. What makes this sonic communion possible is

> that all these physically distinct nervous systems are cut from the same mold, and all are attuned to the same pattern of sound. (Benzon, 2001, p. 43)

Benzon's belief in the evolutionary, biological necessity of social bonding through participation in musical events leads him to a state of alarm concerning the reliance on deeply individual, non-participatory musical experience in so much of contemporary life. He feels, like Freeman, that musical participation is not just a pleasant pastime, but a social necessity. We must all continue to share in each other's bodily rhythms in order to experience our common humanity, in order to promote enterprises for the common good. Singing and dancing together in time with the music may be one of humanity's greatest accomplishments.

ACKNOWLEDGMENTS

I am grateful to my research assistant, Joshua Penman, whose combination of musical, technological, theoretical, and scientific skills were invaluable at every stage of the research project. I am also grateful to Dr. Kathleen Welch, statistical consultant, Center for Statistical Consultation and Research, University of Michigan, and to Sandra Becker, Department of Psychology, for their generous help with the statistical analysis. I also wish to acknowledge the assistance of Dr. Barbara Kamholz, Associate Professor of Psychiatry, Medical School, University of Michigan, for compiling psychological data concerning the various groups. Finally, I wish to thank Pastor Nathaniel Nix of the Pine View Apostolic Faith Church in Ypsilanti, Michigan.

NOTES

1. GSR is recognized as a standard measure of emotional arousal involving the sympathetic branch of the autonomic nervous system (ANS; e.g., Raskin, 1973; Bouscein, 1992; Tarvainenn et al., 2001; Stern et al. Quigley, 2001; Khalfa, Peretz, Blondin, & Mannon, 2002). It is the measurement of a small electrical current between two electrodes attached to the fingertips of the participant. In response to ANS arousal, the moment-to-moment activity of the sweat glands in the hand causes changes in the relative conductance of a small electrical current between the two electrodes.
2. What follows is an abbreviated description of this experiment. For a fuller description, see "Religious Ecstatics, Deep Listeners, and Musical Emotions," *Empirical Musicology Review*, 4(2), 2009.

REFERENCES

Aramaki, S., Kira, Y., & Hirasawa, Y. (1997). A study of the normal values and habituation phenomenon of sympathetic skin response. *American Journal of Physical Medicine and Rehabilitation, 76*, 2–7.

Barthes, R. (1986). Rasch. In R. Howard (Trans.), *The responsibility of forms: Critical essays on music, art, and representation* (pp. 299–312). New York: Hill and Wang.

Becker, J. (2004). *Deep listeners: Music, emotion, and trancing.* Bloomington IN: Indiana University Press.

Benzon, W. L. (2001). *Beethoven's anvil: Music in mind and culture.* New York: Basic Books.

Blood, A. J., & Zatorre, R. J. (2001). Intensely pleasurable responses to music correlate with activity in brain regions implicated in reward and emotion. *Proceedings of the National Academy of Science USA, 98*(20), 11818–11823.

Boucsein, W. (1992). *Electrodermal activity.* New York: Plenum Press.

Clayton, M., Sager, R., & Will, U. (2005). In time with the music: The concept of entrainment and its significance for ethnomusicology. *European Meetings in Ethnomusicology Special Esem-CounterPoint, Vol. 11.*

Clynes, M. (1986). When time is music. In J. Evans & M. Clynes (Eds.), *Rhythm in psychological, linguistic and musical processes* (pp. 169–224). Springfield, IL: Charles C. Thomas.

Condon, W. S. (1986). Communication: Rhythm and structure. In J. Evans & M. Clynes (Eds.), *Rhythm in psychological, linguistic and musical processes* (pp. 55–77). Springfield, IL: C. C. Thomas.

Davis, W. B., & Thaut, M. H. (1989). The influence of preferred relaxing music on measures of state anxiety, relaxation, and physiological responses. *Journal of Music Therapy, 26*(4), 168–187.

Eisenstein, E. M., Eisenstein, D., & Bonheim, P. (1991). Initial habituation or sensitization of the GSR depends on magnitude of first response. *Physiology and Behavior, 49*, 211–215.

Eliot, T. S. (1943). *Four quartets.* New York: Harcourt, Brace.

Erickson, F., & Mohatt, G. (1982). Cultural organization in participation structures in two classrooms of Indian students. In G. Spindler (Ed.), *Doing the ethnography of schooling: Educational anthropology in action* (pp. 132–174). New York: Holt. Rinehart and Winston.

Freeman, W. (2000). A neurobiological role of music in social bonding. In N. L. Wallin, Bjorn Merker, & S. Brown (Eds.), *The origins of music* (pp. 411–424). Cambridge, MA: The MIT Press.

Gabrielsson, A. (2001). Emotions in strong experiences with music. In P. N. Juslin & J. A. Sloboda (Eds.), *Music and emotion: Theory and research* (pp. 431–449). Oxford: Oxford University Press.

Gabrielsson, A., & Lindstrom, S. (1993). On strong experiences of music. *Musik Psychologie, 10*, 118–140.

Gabrielsson, A., & Wik, S. L. (2000). Strong experiences of and with music. In D. Greer (Ed.), *Musicology and sister disciplines: Past, present, future.* Proceedings of the 16th International Congress of the International Musicological Society, London, 1997. Oxford: Oxford University Press.

Haas, F., Distenfeld, S., & Axen, K. (1986). Effects of perceived musical rhythm on respiratory pattern. *Journal of Applied Physiology, 61*(3), 1185–1191.

Harrer, G., & Harrer, H. (1977). Music, emotion and autonomic function. In M. Critchley & R. A. Henson (Eds.), *Music and the brain: Studies in the neurology of music* (pp. 202–216). London: William Heinemann Medical Books Limited.

Hodges, D. E., (Ed.). (1980). *Handbook of music psychology*. Lawrence, KS: National Association for Music Therapy, Inc.

Janata, P., & Grafton, S. T. (2003). Swinging in the brain: Shared neural substrates for behavior related to sequencing and music. *Nature Neuroscience, 6*(7), 682–687.

Janata, P., Tillmann, B., & Bharucha, J. J. (2002). Listening to polyphonic music recruits domain-general attention and working memory circuits. *Cognitive, Affective and Behavioral Neuroscience, 2*, 121–140.

Khalfa, S., Peretz, I., Blondin, J. P., & Manon, R. (2002). Event-related skin conductance responses to musical emotions in humans. *Neuroscience Letters, 328*, 145–149.

Krumhansl, C. L. (1997). An exploratory study of musical emotions and psychophysiology. *Canadian Journal of Experimental Psychology, 51*(4), 336–362.

Large, E. (2001). On synchronizing movements to music. *Human Movement Science, 19*(4), 527–566.

Lerdahl, F., & Jackendoff, R. (1983). *A generative theory of tonal music*. Cambridge, MA: MIT Press.

Maturana, H., & Varela, F. J. (1987). *The tree of knowledge: The biological roots of human understanding*. Boston: New Science Library.

Maxfield, M. (1990). *Effects of rhythmic drumming on EEG and subjective experience* (Doctoral dissertation). San Francisco Institute of Transpersonal Psychology. Cited in P. Wright, Rhythmic drumming in contemporary shamanism and its relationship to auditory driving and risk of seizure precipitation in epileptics, *Anthropology of Consciousness, 2*(34), (1991), 714.

Menon, V., & Levitin, D. J. (2005). The rewards of music listening: Response and physiological connectivity of the mesolimbic system. *NeuroImage, 28*, 175–184.

Merker, B. (2000). Synchronous chorusing and human origins. In N. L. Wallin, B. Merker & S. Brown (Eds.), *The origins of music* (pp. 315–327). Cambridge, MA: The MIT Press.

Meyer, L. (1956). *Emotion and meaning in music*. Chicago: University of Chicago Press.

Miller, M. M., & Strongman, K. T. (2002). The emotional effects of music on religious experience: A study of the Pentecostal-Charismatic style of music and worship. *Psychology of Music, 30*, 8–27.

Neher, A. (1961). Auditory driving observed with scalp electrodes in normal subjects. *Electroencephalography and Clinical Neurophysiology, 13*, 449–451.

Nuñez, R. E. (1997). Eating soup with chopsticks: Dogmas, difficulties and alternatives in the study of conscious experience. *Journal of Consciousness Studies, 4*(2), 143–166.

Oughourlian, J. M. (1991). *The puppet of desire: The psychology of hysteria, possession and hypnosis*. Stanford, CA: Stanford University Press.

Raffman, D. (1993). *Language, music, and mind*. Cambridge: The MIT Press.

Raskin, D. C. (1973). Attention and arousal. In W. F. Prokasy & D. C. Raskin (Eds.), *Electrodermal activity in psychological research* (pp. 125–155). New York and London: Academic Press.

Rickard, N. S. (2004). Intense emotional responses to music: A test of the physiological arousal hypothesis. *Psychology of Music, 32*(4), 371–388.

Rouget, G. (1985). *Music and trance: A theory of the relations between music and possession* (B. Biebuyck, Trans.). Chicago: University of Chicago Press.

Stern, R. M., Ray, W., & Quigley, K. S. (2001). *Psychophysiological recording, 2nd ed*. Oxford: Oxford University Press.

Sylvan, R. (2005). *Trance formation: The spiritual and religious dimensions of global rave culture*. New York, London: Routledge.

Tannen, D. (1984). *Conversational style: Analyzing talk among friends.* Norwood, NJ: Ablex.

Tarvainenn, M. P., Karjalainen, P. A., Koistinen, A. S., Valkonen-Korhonen, M., Partanen, J., & Karjalainen, P. A. (2001). Analysis of galvanic skin responses with principal components and clustering techniques. *IEEE Transactions on Biomedical Engineering, 48*(10), 1071–1078.

Thaut, M. H. (1990). Neuropsychological processes in music perception and their relevance in music therapy. In R. F. Unkefer (Ed.), *Music therapy in the treatment of adults with mental disorders: Theoretical bases and clinical interventions* (pp. 3–32). New York: Schirmer Books.

Thaut, M. H., & Davis, W. B. (1993). The influence of subject-selected versus experimenter-chosen music on affect, anxiety, and relaxation. *Journal of Music Therapy, 30,* 210–233.

Toyokura, M. (1998). Waveform and habituation of sympathetic skin response. *Electroencephalography and Clinical Neurophysiology, 109,* 178–183.

Wallin, N. L. (1991). *Biomusicology: Neurophysiological, neuropsychological, and evolutionary perspectives on the origins and purposes of music.* Stuyvesent, NY: Pendragon Press.

Will, U., & Berg, E. (2007). Brain wave synchronization and entrainment to periodic acoustic stimuli. *Neuroscience Letters, 424,* 55–60.

Witvliet, C.V., & Vrana, S. R. (1995). Psychophysiological responses as indices of affective dimensions. *Psychophysiology, 32*(5), 436–443.

Zakharova, N. N., & Avdeev, V. M. (1982). [Functional changes in the central nervous system during music perception (study of positive emotions)]. *Zh Vyssh Nerv Deiat Im I P Pavlova, 32*(5), 915–924.

Zimny, G. H., & Weidenfeller, E. W. (1963). Effects of music upon GSR and heart rate. *The American Journal of Psychology, 76*(2), 311–314.1.

4   A Scientific View of Musical Rhythm

Matthew Wright

INTRODUCTION

Musical rhythm in general is quite a challenge to measure and describe accurately. This chapter attempts to describe the elements of musical rhythm in scientific terms both to define these elements for the benefit of other portions of the book and also to give an overall sense of the complexity of the topic.

ESTABLISHING TERMS: REPETITION, PERIODICITY, PHASE

Musical *repetition* refers to the perception that something discrete keeps happening at regular time intervals, for example, a dripping faucet. The same repetition could be called *periodicity* when we perceive that an overall shape keeps repeating without there necessarily being a clear beginning and ending point, like the up and down pitch of a siren. The only difference is in how we think of the unit that repeats.

Much of the theory of mathematics and signal processing is based on the ideal of exact repetition. For example, an *oscillator* is an abstract mathematical tool that cycles through a repeating pattern; Figure 4.1 can be interpreted as the output of a sine wave oscillator. A *period* is the amount of time that an oscillator takes to go through its repeating pattern one time, in this case, one second. The *phase* of a signal, at any given time, is its proportion of the way through the period at that time; the bottom graph in Figure 4.1 shows the phase as a function of time. *Frequency* is the rate of repetition, in other words the reciprocal of period; it is also the rate of phase change.[1]

We can bring together musical and mathematical terminology by using an oscillator as a model of an ideal metronome. It "ticks" when the phase is zero, and the frequency is proportional to the tempo.[2] The period is the duration of one beat. The current phase is the proportion of time that has elapsed between the previous tick and the next tick.

As an example of *phase relationships*, imagine two ideal metronomes set to the exact same tempo. If they start at exactly the same time, they

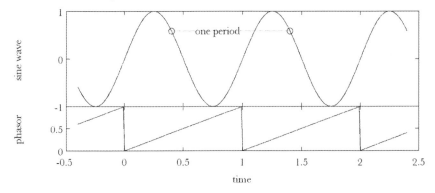

Figure 4.1   Example of an ideal sine wave oscillator.

will always tick at exactly the same time infinitely into the future. In this case we say the oscillators are *in phase* with each other; that is, their phase difference is zero. If the metronome on the left starts first, and then the metronome on the right starts exactly halfway between the ticks of the metronome on the left, so that they alternate evenly "left, right, left, right" then we say they are exactly *out of phase* with each other; that is, their phase difference is 0.5.[3] A phase difference of 0.1 would mean that the second metronome always ticks 10% of the way between the first metronome's ticks, etc.

Perception of repetition is qualitatively different depending on the period. One very important length of time for human perception is the *perceptual present*, lasting 2–6 seconds; this is the amount of time a sound can be stored in short-term memory without necessitating long-term memory recall (E. F. Clarke, 1999). Beyond the perceptual present, we notice repetition only by comparing new input to our memory, whereas within the perceptual present we "automatically" perceive repetition in terms of rhythm. Another important length of time is around 50ms: repetition faster than this starts to sound like a musical tone rather than a series of discrete sounds, engaging our perception of pitch rather than of rhythm.

Of course there is no perfectly exact repetition in the musical world. Any quasi-repeating sound produced by human activity will have small "errors" in timing caused by what is known as "motor noise"; these are never much less than about 1 millisecond and often much more.[4] Only mechanical means such as tape loops and their digital equivalents can produce repetition that is exact to within the limits of human perception, and indeed a lot of popular music and the vast majority of electronic dance music is constructed digitally with exact repetition of rhythmic sequences or of a segment of prerecorded audio. Likewise, many of the synthetic stimuli used to probe rhythmic perception experimentally consist of inhumanly perfect repetition of sound.

ESTABLISHING WHEN A MUSICAL EVENT OCCURS IS HARDER THAN IT SOUNDS: GROUND TRUTH

It is often useful to conceptualize sound as consisting of independent, distinct *events* (for example, musical notes). It is useful because many sounds are indeed produced by distinct, all-or-nothing physical actions, for example, striking, plucking, dropping, plosive consonants, etc. Many other sounds are produced by continuous physical actions, for example, vowels, voiced consonants, wind, crumpling, a vibrating reed, bowing, scraping, etc., and even in these cases the notion of a discrete event (for example, the beginning, a change of state, arrival at a quasi-steady value) is often a good match to human perception and therefore very useful.[5] The fascinating question of how our minds organize perceived sound into these discrete events is one aspect of *auditory scene analysis* (Bregman, 1990).

The subjectivity in the perception of discrete musical events manifests as difficulties in trying to establish perceptual "ground truth" from human listeners.[6] For example, Leveau, Daudet, and Richard each hand-labeled the beginning times of all of the discrete musical events in 17 short musical excerpts (6 to 30 seconds) in a variety of musical styles. Even though they all used the same software tool to perform the labeling, which they had themselves written, they often disagreed not only on the exact timing of the events, but also on the number of events in the excerpt. (Leveau, Daudet, & Richard, 2004). Tanghe et al. came across the same problem trying to get expert percussionists to mark all discrete drum events in various recordings:

> Brushes for example have a typical 'dragged' sound which is hard to annotate as a single percussive event. In this case most annotators chose to register the accents of the brush sounds. Snare rolls do consist of a series of discernable percussive onsets, but it's very hard to annotate the many fast strokes accurately. The same is true for 'flammed' drums (typically the snare drum) where two hits of the same drum type are deliberately played almost (but not quite) at the same time, leading to the sensation of a ghost note occurring slightly before a main note. (Tanghe et al., 2005, p. 54)

PERCEPTUAL ONSET AND PERCEPTUAL ATTACK TIME

Physical onset is the actual acoustic beginning of a sound event, that is, the moment that the event's amplitude first becomes greater than zero. For synthesized sound, it is easy to say when the amplitude first becomes nonzero. For recorded acoustic sound there is always a noise floor, and so there is always some ambiguity and/or subjectivity in choosing the instant that the event's amplitude first rises above the noise floor. The *perceptual onset* is the moment at which a listener can first hear that an event has begun (Vos & Rasch, 1981).

A musical event's *Perceptual Attack Time* ("PAT") is its perceived moment of rhythmic placement (Gordon, 1987; Collins, 2006; Wright, 2008).[7] Note that whereas physical onset is an aspect of the signal itself, the perceptual onset and perceptual attack time are subjective, perceptual parameters.

For highly percussive sounds, the perceptual onset might be the same as the physical onset time, and the PAT might also be the same, or just a few milliseconds later. However, for sounds with a slow attack, for example, bowed violin, the PAT might be dozens of milliseconds after the physical onset. My own model of PAT treats it not as a discrete instant but rather as a probability density function (Wright, 2008); my results supported the hypothesis that the variance of a sound's measured PAT depends both on the degree of percussiveness of the sound and also on the degree of spectral similarity to the reference sound by which it is being judged.

Figure 4.2 illustrates these three moments for a hypothetical sound event: time zero is defined as the time of the physical onset, the perceptual onset comes shortly later, the PAT is yet later, and the amplitude/energy maximum is even later. The *transient* at the beginning of a sound event is the segment of time starting at the physical onset and lasting until the sound achieves some kind of steady state. There may be other transients later in a sound event and especially at the end. Here is another definition: "As a preliminary informal definition, transients are short intervals during which the signal evolves quickly in some nontrivial or relatively unpredictable way" (Bello et al., 2005, p. 1036). Any detailed empirical study of musicians' timing, whether alone or in groups, must take PAT into account, especially when choosing stimuli and analyzing the response data.

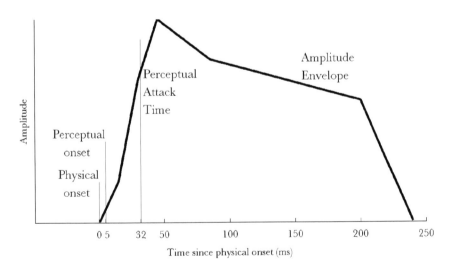

Figure 4.2 Amplitude envelope of a hypothetical sound, displaying hypothetical physical and perceptual onsets and perceptual attack time.

LEARNING

Figure 4.3 depicts the main feedback loop in the process of learning to play music. This is what might be called the "forward model," in which we assume that the musician starts with an idea of what sound to make ("intention").[8] The brain translates these into nervous system messages that propagate to various muscles ("motor control"), causing them to contract in varying degrees as functions of time ("body") so as to control a musical instrument ("instrument").[9] This then produces a sound (or not), to which the musician listens[10] ("perception"). Some part of the brain then compares what the musician perceives to what was intended. The gap between intent and perception then drives the learning process, as the musician consciously and unconsciously adapts[11] the mapping from intention to motor control.

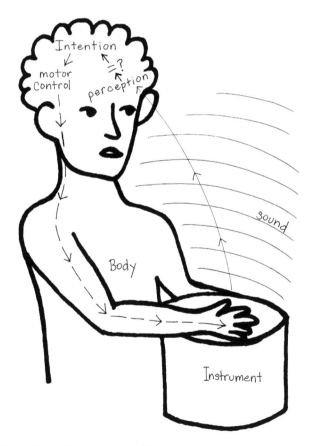

Figure 4.3   The primary feedback loop in learning to play music (drawn by Michelle Logan).

PAT is an integral part of the "perception" link, and therefore part of the entire feedback loop. There are already tens or hundreds of milliseconds of lag time between when the brain issues motor control commands and when the body actually produces sound, due to the slowness of chemical message propagation in the nervous system, the body's and instrument's inertia, and other physical considerations. Our brains are very good at generating motor commands the appropriate amount of time before we want an action to take effect, and at fine-tuning these kinds of time relationships when learning various physical activities.

Therefore a violinist, for example, has learned to time her motor behavior so that notes' perceptual attack times follow the desired rhythm, not the notes' physical onsets. The delay between a note's onset and its PAT is just another lag that the brain learns to compensate for; that is why, for example, pipe organists can learn to play accurate rhythms even when there are hundreds or thousands of milliseconds of delay between pressing a key and hearing the corresponding note.

PULSATION, MICROTIMING, AND METER

Pulsation is a regular series of instants that are possible event attack times. Each pulse can be thought of as a container that holds either the PAT of an event or not, that is, only some of the pulses have notes. In the ideal (a.k.a. "metronomic") case, the pulses are perfectly regular, and each sound's attack time coincides precisely with one of the pulses. In the real-world case of music performed expressively by human beings there are two complicating factors (Honing, 2001; Iyer, Bilmes, Wessel, & Wright, 1997; Palmer, 1997), known collectively as *microtiming*:

1. The series of pulses is not exactly regular, but instead the frequency changes slowly as a function of time. These *tempo curves* (Desain & Honing, 1992b; Honing, 2001) have been studied and modeled extensively for modern-day performance practice of European music of the Classical and Romantic periods (Todd, 1995; Widmer & Goebl, 2004); they're generally correlated to the phrase structure that the performer wants to bring out. Many researchers have also charted the variation of tempo in recordings of non-Western music (Bilmes, 1993; Clayton, 2000; Clayton, Sager, & Will, 2004, p. 29; Schloss, 1985; Tzanetakis, Kapur, Schloss, & Wright, 2007).
2. Each event's attack time does not exactly coincide with the time of a pulse, but instead may be early or late by tens of milliseconds. This "asynchrony" or "deviation" might form a regular repeating pattern as in Jazz "swing" (Collier & Collier, 2002; Dixon, Gouyon, & Widmer, 2004; Friberg & Sundstroöm, 1997; Friberg & Sundström,

1999, 2002; Gouyon, Fabig, & Bonada, 2003; Lindsay, 2006; Lindsay & Nordquist, 2006, 2007; Waadeland, 2001, 2003) or Brazilian "swingee" (Lindsay, 2006; Lindsay & Nordquist, 2006, 2007; Wright & Berdahl, 2006), "systematic variation" of note durations in, for example, Viennese Waltz or Swedish folk tunes (Gabrielsson, 1982), or Clynes' controversial "composer's pulse" (Clynes, 1983) for historical Western composers. In addition, each individual note might have its own deviation from the time of the pulse for reasons including accentuation or differentiation from other instruments, etc. (Iyer, 1998). In addition to these intentional asynchronies, motor noise also adds at least 1 ms of random jitter to each note's attack time even for the most skilled performers.

Meter (London, 2004) involves pulsation no faster than about 100 ms (the psychological limit on perceiving very fast distinct events) and no slower than about 6 seconds (the duration of the "perceptual present"). Meter requires at least two levels of pulsation (also called *metric levels*) at different rates, with well-defined phase and frequency relationships among all levels; in other words a single stream of pulses is not in itself meter. The "main" or most salient metric level is the *beat* or *tactus*, and is usually defined as the metric level to which most listeners will tap their feet.

PHRASING

Phrasing is the perceived connection among discrete events that occur nearby in time, usually together within the perceptual present.[12] One question is how our minds group perceived events into phrases. Lerdahl's and Jackendoff's *Generative Theory of Tonal Music* includes many rules for grouping musical notes together into phrases (Lerdahl & Jackendoff, 1983). Bregman has another set of rules for grouping events into auditory streams (Bregman, 1990). Todd's "rhythmogram" (Todd, 1994) is a graphical representation of musical material that brings out grouping structure. Rothstein's "tonal phrases" require harmonic motion by definition (Rothstein, 1989).

Saying which groups of events "group" together is only part of the story about phrasing; There are also musical parameters that vary over certain shapes across entire phrases. For example, most attempts at computer-generated stylistically correct renditions of piano music vary the tempo systematically over the course of each musical phrase (Friberg, 1995; Sundberg, Askenfelt, & Frydén, 1983; Sundberg, Friberg, & Bresin, 2003; Widmer, 2002; Widmer & Goebl, 2004). Bilmes' system for machine learning of microtiming in the Afro-Cuban rumba genre used a sophisticated form of lookup based on the assumption that similar phrases will have similar microtiming (Bilmes, 1993).

PREDICTION

Finally, I want to emphasize the role of prediction by listeners (and performers) in musical rhythm. Our brains do not just wait passively for information to trickle up through the auditory nerve and form events, phrases, meter, and other structure; they actively predict what we will hear through top-down models as well as these bottom-up processes (Slaney, 1997). Hawkins goes so far as to define intelligence completely in terms of prediction (Hawkins & Blakeslee, 2004). There are just as many nerves running from our brains back to our ears as in the other direction, and the cochlea is not just a passive encoder of incoming sound, but a nonlinear active system with feedback, giving us increased frequency and amplitude resolution perhaps by fine-tuning the mechanics to focus on what we expect to hear (Zwicker & Fastl, 1999).

David Huron has proposed a wide-reaching model of expectation that illuminates many aspects of music (Huron, 2006). Mari Reiss Jones suggested that the ability to pay attention to incoming sound is a limited quantity, and proposed a nonlinear oscillator model that uses meter to predict when new events will occur so as to best utilize these attentional resources (Large & Jones, 1999). Even the simple delay lines in Scheirer's beat tracker can be interpreted as a form of prediction of what sound will come in the future (Scheirer, 1998, p. 593).

Snyder and Large were able to measure metric prediction in the brain's gamma-band activity via an EEG (Snyder & Large, 2005). Subjects heard an isochronous sequence of synthetic stimuli with some of the events randomly omitted. Whereas *evoked* gamma band activity depended on whether or not the subject had heard an event, *induced* gamma band activity began *before* the expected time of the event and increased up to that time, even in cases where no event actually sounded.

CONCLUSION

There is more to musical rhythm than one may think, and these complexities could be important in research protocols concerning the study of rhythm. As I hope this chapter has demonstrated, musical rhythm consists of much more than exact repetition, so experiments measuring responses to such mechanical stimuli cannot give us the whole story about the effect of musical rhythm on the human brain. Repetition at different time scales produces qualitatively distinct perceptual effects and these must also be carefully considered.

The issue of physical onset versus perceptual onset versus perceptual attack time could be important when studying evoked potentials: a sound with an onset far before the PAT could evoke a different brain response than a sound that peaks soon after the attack. Indeed, the PAT, though much more difficult to quantify than the onset, may be the preferred way to consider the timing of rhythmic stimuli in such experiments. Likewise, a participant's subjective grouping of stimuli (e.g., according to meter and/or phrasing) may very well determine brain response data; this must also be considered carefully in experimental design.

NOTES

1. Frequency in Hertz is the rate of phase change when phase is defined to go from 0 to 1 (as is the usual convention when discussing phase in the context of musical rhythm). If phase goes from 0 to 2π then radian frequency (which is 2π times frequency in Hertz) is the rate of phase change.
2. Musical tempo is usually measured in beats per minute ("BPM"); divide this by 60 to get beats per second, which is the frequency of the metronome in Hertz.
3. Again, I'm using the convention of phase from 0 to 1. "Exactly out of phase" would correspond to a phase difference of "180 degrees" or "pi radians."
4. This motor noise turns out to be difficult to measure. One method is to ask subjects to tap at a variety of steady frequencies and measure the variance, then decompose this variance into a "central clock variance," i.e., the mind's inability to maintain a perfectly steady tempo, plus the motor noise as an added source of variance (Wing & Kristofferson, 1973a, 1973b). With these methods, "typically the motor variance is in the range of about 25 ms-squared (i.e., standard deviation of about 5 ms) and changes little with tempo" (Bruno Repp, personal communication, January 31, 2008). Rubine and McAvinney put this figure around 1.5 to 4ms (Rubine & McAvinney, 1990), whereas Desain and Honing say 10–100 ms (Desain, Honing, & Rijk, 1989), both citing (Vorberg & Hambuch, 1978). See also (Lago & Kon, 2004). Another method is to ask a performer to play a piece "the same way" two or more times and then measure the correlation in note durations among the results (Repp, 1995). This approach also suffers from the methodological problem of separating the mind's variance from the body's.
5. The danger arises from adopting a worldview in which all music a priori consists of discrete events. Western music notation, the MIDI protocol (Moore, 1988), and most music software support this worldview by providing notes and other events as primitives. However, musical meaning and even rhythm can also be conveyed by continuous shapes of time with no clear division into distinct events.
6. The phrase "ground truth" comes originally from analysis of aerial photographs and satellite imagery, in which conclusions drawn from such images are double-checked by information collected on site, in other words, on the ground. The term has made its way into the jargon of machine learning to refer more broadly to any data for which the correct "answers" are known.
7. Perceptual Center or P-center (or P-centre) is the corresponding concept to PAT in the relatively vast literature on speech, where the discrete event is a syllable (Harsin, 1997; Howell, 1988a, 1988b; Janker, 1995, 1996; Marcus, 1981; Morton, Marcus, & Frankish, 1976; Patel, Lofqvist, & Naito, 1999; Rapp-Holmgren, 1971; Scott, 1998; Soraghan, Ward, Villing, & Timoney, 2005; Villing, Ward, & Timoney, 2003, 2007; Vos, Mates, & Kruysbergen, 1995).
8. A more complete model would take into account the very important exploratory aspects of discovering sounds that can be produced. There can be a sense of discovering the possibilities of an instrument in an acoustic space,

rather than a predefined sonic goal to reproduce. Whatever the sources and dynamics of the musician's intention, the rest of the feedback loop works as described here.

9. Here the term "instrument" includes the human voice, clapping, etc.
10. Depending on the instrument, the musician might also feel the effects of touching the instrument, see the instrument, or, in principle, smell or taste it. Visual and haptic feedback are optional, yet sometimes very important, aspects of musical instruments, and when present they are part of this feedback loop. I believe that predominantly a musician's intention is an idea of what sound he or she wants to produce, though in many interesting cases music is organized (at least in performers' minds) according to the body's movement patterns on a particular instrument; see Baily, 1991.
11. The musician's body itself also adapts as a result of practice, e.g., guitarist's calluses, wind players' strong embouchures, etc.
12. The term "phrase" can also refer to a grammatical unit. Musical phrases are related to spoken phrases: For example, the prosody that organizes the words of a spoken sentence to clarify the meaning uses the musical parameters of pitch and timing.

REFERENCES

Baily, J. (1991). Some cognitive aspects of motor planning in musical performance. *Psychologica Belgica, 31*(2), 147–162.
Bello, J. P., Daudet, L., Abdallah, S., Duxbury, C., Davies, M., & Sandler, M. B. (2005). A tutorial on onset detection in music signals. *IEEE Transactions on Speech and Audio Processing, 13*(5), 1035–1047.
Bilmes, J. (1993). *Timing is of the essence: Perceptual and computational techniques for representing, learning, and reproducing timing in percussive rhythm.* Unpublished Master's thesis. Massachusetts Institute of Technology, Cambridge, MA.
Bregman, A. S. (1990). *Auditory scene analysis: The perceptual organization of sound.* Cambridge, MA: MIT Press.
Clarke, E. F. (1999). Rhythm and timing in music. In D. Deutsch (Ed.), *The Psychology of Music* (pp. 473–500). San Diego: Academic Press.
Clayton, M. (2000). *Time in Indian music: Rhythm, metre, and form in North Indian Râg performance.* Oxford: Oxford University Press.
Clayton, M., Sager, R., & Will, U. (2004). In time with the music: The concept of entrainment and its significance for ethnomusicology. *ESEM CounterPoint, 1,* 1–45.
Clynes, M. (1983). Expressive microstructure in music, linked to living qualities. In J. Sundberg (Ed.), *Studies of music performance* (pp. 76–181). Stockholm: Royal Swedish Academy of Music.
Collier, G. L., & Collier, J. L. C. (2002). A study of timing in two Louis Armstrong solos. *Music Perception, 19*(3), 463–483.
Collins, N. (2006). *Investigating computational models of perceptual attack time.* Paper presented at the 9th International Conference on Music Perception and Cognition, Bologna.
Desain, P., & Honing, H. (1992). Tempo curves considered harmful. In P. Desain & H. Honing (Eds.), *Music, mind, and machine* (pp. 25–40). Amsterdam: Thesis Publishers.
Desain, P., Honing, H. & Rijk, K.de. (1989). The Quantization of Musical Time: A Connectionist Approach, *Computer Music Journal 13(3),* (pp. 150–167). Amsterdam: Thesis Publishers.

Dixon, S., Gouyon, F., & Widmer, G. (2004). *Towards characterisation of music via rhythmic patterns.* Paper presented at the 5th International Conference on Music Information Retrieval (ISMIR), Barcelona.

Friberg, A. (1995). *Matching the rule parameters of Phrase Arch to performances of "Träumerei:" A preliminary study.* Paper presented at the KTH Symposion on Grammars for Music Performance, Stockholm, Sweden.

Friberg, A., & Sundström, A. (1999). Jazz drummers' swing ratio in relation to tempo. *Journal of the Acoustical Society of America, 105*(2), 1330 (abstract only).

Friberg, A., & Sundström, A. (2002). Swing ratios and ensemble timing in jazz performance: Evidence for a common rhythmic pattern. *Music Perception, 19*(3), 333–349.

Friberg, A., & Sundstroöm, A. (1997). Preferred swing ratio in jazz as a function of tempo. *Speech Music and Hearing Quarterly Progress and Status Report,* April, 19–28.

Gabrielsson, A. (1982). Perception and performance of musical rhythm. In M. Clynes (Ed.), *Music, mind, and brain: The neuropsychology of music* (pp. 159–169). New York: Plenum Press.

Gordon, J. W. (1987). The perceptual attack time of musical tones. *Journal of the Acoustical Society of America, 82*(1), 88–105.

Gouyon, F., Fabig, L., & Bonada, J. (2003). *Rhythmic expressiveness transformations of audio recordings: Swing modifications.* Paper presented at the 6th International Conference on Digital Audio Effects (DAFx 03), London.

Harsin, C. A. (1997). Perceptual-center modeling is affected by including acoustic rate-of-change modulations. *Perception and Psychophysics, 59*(2), 243–251.

Hawkins, J., & Blakeslee, S. (2004). *On intelligence: How a new understanding of the brain will lead to the creation of truly intelligent machines.* New York: Owl Books/Henry Holt and Company.

Honing, H. (2001). From time to time: The representation of timing and tempo. *Computer Music Journal, 25*(3), 50–61.

Howell, P. (1988a). Prediction of P-center location from the distribution of energy in the amplitude envelope: I. *Perception and Psychophysics, 43,* 99.

Howell, P. (1988b). Prediction of P-center location from the distribution of energy in the amplitude envelope: II. *Perception and Psychophysics, 43,* 90–93.

Huron, D. (2006). *Sweet anticipation: Music and the psychology of expectation.* Cambridge, MA: MIT Press.

Iyer, V. (1998). *Microstructures of feel, macrostructures of sound: Embodied cognition in West African and African-American musics.* Unpublished Ph.D. thesis. University of California at Berkeley, Berkeley.

Iyer, V., Bilmes, J., Wessel, D. L., & Wright, M. (1997). *A novel representation for rhythmic structure.* Paper presented at the International Computer Music Conference, Thessaloniki, Hellas.

Janker, P. M. (1995). *On the influence of the internal structure of a syllable on the P-center-perception.* Paper presented at the 13th International Congress of Phonetic Sciences, Stockholm.

Janker, P. M. (1996). Evidence for the P-center syllable-nucleus-onset correspondence hypothesis. *Zaspil (ZAS Papers in Linguistics), 7,* 94–124.

Lago, N. P., & Kon, F. (2004). *The quest for low latency.* Paper presented at the International Computer Music Conference, Miami, FL.

Large, E. W., & Jones, M. R. (1999). The dynamics of attending: How people track time-varying events. *Psychological Review, 106*(1), 119–159.

Lerdahl, F., & Jackendoff, R. (1983). *A generative theory of tonal music.* Cambridge, Mass: MIT Press.

Leveau, P., Daudet, L., & Richard, G. (2004). *Methodology and tools for the evaluation of automatic onset detection algorithms in music.* Paper presented at the

5th Annual International Conference on Music Information Retrieval (ISMIR), Barcelona.

Lindsay, K. A. (2006). *Rhythm analyzer: A technical look at swing rhythm in music.* Unpublished Master's thesis. Southern Oregon University, Ashland, OR.

Lindsay, K. A., & Nordquist, P. R. (2006). A technical look at swing rhythm in music. *Journal of Acoustical Society of America, 120*(5), 3005 (abstract only).

Lindsay, K. A., & Nordquist, P. R. (2007). More than a feeling—Some technical details of swing rhythm in music. *Acoustics Today,* July, 2007, 31–42.

London, J. (2004). *Hearing in Time: Psychological Aspects of Musical Meter.* Oxford: Oxford University Press.

Marcus, S. M. (1981). Acoustic determinants of perceptual center (P-center) location. *Perception and Psychophysics, 30*(3), 247–256.

Morton, J., Marcus, S., & Frankish, C. (1976). Theoretical note: Perceptual centers (P-centers). *Psychological Review, 83*(5), 405–408.

Moore, F. R. (1988). The Dysfunctions of MIDI. *Computer Music Journal, 12*(1), 19–28.

Palmer, C. (1997). Music performance. *Annual Review of Psychology, 48,* 115–138.

Patel, A. D., Lofqvist, A., & Naito, W. (1999). *The acoustics and kinematics of regularly timed speech: A database and method for the study of the P-Center problem.* Paper presented at the 14th International Congress of Phonetic Sciences, San Fransisco, CA.

Rapp-Holmgren, K. (1971). *A study of syllable timing.* KTH Department for Speech, Music, and Hearing Quarterly Progress and Status Report, 1–19.

Repp, B. H. (1995). Expressive timing in Schumann's "Träumerei:"' An analysis of performances by graduate student pianists. *Journal of the Acoustical Society of America, 98*(5), 2413–2427.

Rothstein, W. (1989). *Phrase rhythm in tonal music.* New York: Schirmer Books.

Rubine, D., & McAvinney, P. (1990). Programmable finger-tracking instrument controllers. *Computer Music Journal, 14*(1), 26–41.

Scheirer, E. D. (1998). Tempo and beat analysis of acoustic musical signals. *Journal of the Acoustical Society of America, 103*(1), 588–601.

Schloss, W. A. (1985). *On the automatic transcription of percussive music: From acoustic signal to high-level analysis.* Unpublished Ph.D. dissertation. Stanford, Palo Alto, CA.

Scott, S. (1998). The point of P-centres. *Psychological Research, 61*(1), 4–11.

Slaney, M. (1997). A critique of pure audition. In D. Rosenthal & H. Okuno (Eds.), *Computational auditory scene analysis* (pp. 27–42). Mahwah, NJ: Lawrence Erlbaum Associates.

Snyder, J. S., & Large, E. W. (2005). Gamma-band activity reflects the metric structure of rhythmic tone sequences. *Cognitive Brain Research, 24,* 117–126.

Soraghan, C. J., Ward, T. E., Villing, R., & Timoney, J. (2005). *Perceptual centre correlates in evoked potentials.* Paper presented at the 3rd European Medical and Biological Engineering Conference (EMBEC 05), Prague.

Sundberg, J., Askenfelt, A., & Frydén, L. (1983). Musical performance. A synthesis-by-rule approach. *Computer Music Journal, 7,* 37–43.

Sundberg, J., Friberg, A., & Bresin, R. (2003). Attempts to reproduce a pianist's expressive timing with Director Musices performance rules. *Journal of New Music Research, 32*(3), 317–325.

Tanghe, K., Lesaffre, M., Degroeve, S., Leman, M., Baets, B. D., & Martens, J.-P. (2005). *Collecting ground truth annotations for drum detection in polyphonic music.* Paper presented at the 6th International Conference on Music Information Retrieval (ISMIR), University of London, London.

Todd, N. P. M. (1994). The auditory "Primal Sketch": A multiscale model of rhythmic grouping. *Journal of New Music Research, 23*(1), 25–70.

Todd, N. P. M. (1995). The kinematics of musical expression. *Journal of the Acoustical Society of America, 97*(3), 1940–1949.

Tzanetakis, G., Kapur, A., Schloss, W. A., & Wright, M. (2007). Computational ethnomusicology. *Journal of Interdisciplinary Music Studies, 1*(2), 1–24.

Villing, R., Ward, T., & Timoney, J. (2003). *P-centre extraction from speech: The need for a more reliable measure.* Paper presented at the Irish Signals and Systems Conference.

Villing, R., Ward, T., & Timoney, J. (2007). *A review of P-Centre models.* Paper presented at the Rhythm Perception and Production Workshop (RPPW), Limerick. http://eprints.nuim.ie/1432/1/TWrppw2007_models_2007b.pdf

Vorberg, D., & Hambuch, R. (1978). On the temporal control of rhythmic performance. In J. Requin (Ed.), *Attention and performance.* Hillsdale, NJ: Lawrence Erlbaum Associates, 535–555.

Vos, J., & Rasch, R. (1981). The perceptual onset of musical tones. *Perception and Psychophysics, 29*(4), 323–335.

Vos, P. G., Mates, J., & Kruysbergen, N. W. V. (1995). The perceptual centre of a stimulus as the cue for synchronization to a metronome: Evidence from asynchronies. *The Quarterly Journal of Experimental Psychology*, Section A, *48*(4), 1024–1040.

Waadeland, C. H. (2001). It don't mean a thing if it ain't got that swing—Simulating expressive timing by modulated movements. *Journal of New Music Research, 30*(1), 23–37.

Waadeland, C. H. (2003). *Analysis of jazz drummers' movements in performance of swing grooves—A preliminary report.* Paper presented at the Stockholm Music Acoustics Conference (SMAC), Stockholm, Sweden, August 6–9.

Widmer, G. (2002). Machine discoveries: A few simple, robust local expression principles. *Journal of New Music Research, 31*(1), 37–50.

Widmer, G., & Goebl, W. (2004). Computational models of expressive music performance: The state of the art. *Journal of New Music Research, 33*(3), 203–216.

Wing, A. M., & Kristofferson, A. B. (1973a). Response delays and the timing of discrete motor responses. *Perception and Psychophysics, 14*, 5–12.

Wing, A. M., & Kristofferson, A. B. (1973b). The timing of interresponse intervals. *Perception and Psychophysics, 13*(3), 455–460.

Wright, M. (2008). The Shape Of an Instant: Measuring and Modeling Perceptual Attack Time with Probability Density Functions. Ph.D. Dissertation. Stanford University.

Wright, M., & Berdahl, E. J. (2006). *Towards machine learning of expressive microtiming in Brazilian drumming.* Paper presented at the International Computer Music Conference, New Orleans, LA.

Zwicker, E., & Fastl, H. (eds.) (1999). Information processing in the auditory system. In *Psychoacoustics: Facts and models* (2nd ed., pp. 23–60). Berlin: Springer.

5 EEG Research Methodology and Brainwave Entrainment

Udo Will and Scott Makeig

PART I. AN INTRODUCTION TO INDEPENDENT COMPONENT
ANALYSIS IN THE STUDY OF MUSIC COGNITION
(SCOTT MAKEIG)

By taking advantage of the new metabolic and hemodynamic imaging modalities, principally Positron Emission Tomography (PET) and functional magnetic resonance imaging (fMRI), brain imaging of music cognition, perception, and production has made notable progress in the last decades (Peretz, Zatorre, 2005). Yet these imaging modalities share a weakness: They each measure only slow, multi-second scale changes in neural activity via indirect measures, whereas music and musical cognition occurs simultaneously on a wide range of time scales, with relatively fast, sub-second sequences of events dominating. To truly observe the brain dynamics supporting musical cognition, therefore, quicker imaging methods are needed. The clear method of choice should be electroencephalography (EEG). EEG captures a more direct measure of neural activity, potential fluctuations that reach the scalp via nearly delay-free volume conduction of spontaneously appearing, locally near-synchronous activities in patches of cortical brain tissue (Freeman Barrie, 2000; Beggs Plenz, 2003).

Yet nearly all EEG studies of music cognition have been handicapped by the limited and restrictive selection of methods used to analyze the recorded data (Makeig et al., 2002, 2004). These have largely been limited to time-domain averaging of recorded EEG epochs time-locked to pre-determined classes of events (for example, standard beeps versus less frequent boops). This response averaging is an ideal method for revealing a fixed brain response buried in noise, for example the small, immediate auditory brainstem response to click stimuli (Galambos Despland, 1980). By 20–150ms after onset of tone stimuli, however, the statistics of the much larger ongoing EEG activity in many parts of the brain have been perturbed in complex ways.

Here, response averaging fails to reveal a single series of response features that can be traced to a fixed sequence of activated brain areas. Rather, response averaging collapses the rich complexity of the data into a few peaks that may bear little resemblance to the mean responses, even, in single cortical areas. Thus, response averaging of scalp-channel EEG data is not an effective method for reducing the spatial complexity inherent in nearly all EEG signals, and does not allow the richness of the EEG brain dynamics accompanying and supporting musical cognition to be well observed or appreciated.

The 1997 PNAS paper we authored (Makeig et al., 1997) was the first journal publication by me and collaborators at Salk Institute, La Jolla of an original approach to EEG decomposition based on the elegant paper by Tony Bell and Terry Sejnowski (1996) on a then-new approach to linear decomposition of independent signals mixed at a number of sensors. The model paradigm was the cocktail party problem: Given a number of microphones all recording a jumble of cocktail party noise, separately extract from their joint data the voices of individual participants as well as any other present sound sources. Furthermore, do this blind, that is, without knowing in advance the nature of the sound sources contributing to the data.

The new idea, first promoted by French applied mathematicians Herault and Jutten (Jutten & Herault, 1991), was that in every case, the actual sound sources could be considered the only sources of distinct information in the data, anything else being their linear mixtures. Therefore, by reversing the mixing process that occurred at the microphones, the recorded sound sources could be unmixed and separated from the data, a process known as independent component analysis (ICA). Tony Bell's elegant Infomax ICA algorithm has proven to be the most stable and reliable approach to ICA for many types of data. Upon reading a pre-print of this paper, one night in 1995, it occurred to me that the same situation and type of result should apply to EEG data. A week later I, with Tony, Terry, and my postdoctoral fellow Tzyy-Ping Jung, submitted a first NIPS conference paper on the success of our very first decomposition (Makeig et al., 1996).

Now, nearly 13 years and many papers later,[1] ICA decomposition is a part of a new approach to signal processing in general, one that may be called information-based signal processing. ICA and a host of related approaches are being applied to data in a huge range of application areas including music decomposition itself (Dubnov Ben-Shalom, 2003). Our first journal article, reprinted here, was published after a long struggle with an obstinate anonymous reviewer at another journal (a world-famous EEG expert, according to the editor) who seemed incapable and/or unwilling to understand the new concept of independence-based decomposition. The ICA approach, and the many further advances it made possible and required, is still judged to be controversial by the many established experts on the simpler EEG response-averaging approach.

Yet, for me and my colleagues, and the hundreds of researchers around the world now using the related open source EEGLAB signal processing environment that I and Arnaud Delorme, with many other contributors, developed and now distribute on the Internet (Delorme & Makeig, 2004), the advantages of the ICA approach to spatial separation of EEG data into distinct sources are becoming ever more apparent.

This first (1997) paper simply re-analyzed average responses time-locked to interruptions in steady-state trains of clicks, presented at a rate near 40/s to one subject, data I had on hand from a previous study. Here, ICA separated three major components of the auditory steady-state response (SSR; Galambos, Makeig, & Talmachoff, 1991). In hindsight, I later realized, the largest of these component processes (ICA-8) was undoubtedly post-auricular muscle activity stimulated by the loud buzzing stimulus—a first, though unwitting example of the now prevalent use of ICA to separate brain and non-brain activities mixed in EEG data. I found this by (later) applying standard equivalent dipole source analysis (Oostenveld Oostendorp, 2002) to the component map, the result being consistent with the location and orientation of post-auricular muscle. This paper thus stands as a caution to scientists looking through new windows into their data: *Do not believe you can immediately understand everything your new window exposes!*

Yet now, 13 years later, the promise of these early results for separating human brain responses to and processing during music listening or production is still nearly unrealized. I, of course, have excuses for my own lack of further progress in this direction. The techniques necessary to handle the complexity of the challenges that moment-to-moment variations in and evolution of a piece of music pose to our brains go quite beyond ICA decomposition. This constant variation and evolution is the essence of music's ability to capture and retain our heartfelt interest, but simple averaging methods (at any level) cannot model the complex relationship between musical events in their individual musical context and EEG dynamic events (in their complex physiological context). The goal and promise of future EEG studies, therefore, is to observe and model the sequence of human brain responses to the challenge of each musical moment, as the listener hears and the performers perform.

I have some new ideas in this direction, however, and have been looking for an interested collaborator who knows enough music and music theory, applied mathematics, and neuroscience to attempt a serious approach to understanding how the brain supports our musical cognition. It is possible I have now met such a person (at the symposiums that led to creation of this book). Let's see what we, and/or others, can accomplish in this direction in coming years!

PART II. EEG RESPONSES TO PERIODIC AUDITORY STIMULI AND BRAINWAVE ENTRAINMENT (UDO WILL)

Introduction

Rhythmic sensorimotor synchronization has received considerable attention in research for over a century (Stetson, 1905; Stevens, 1886). Though finger tapping seems to be the preferred object of study, other limb move-ments have also been investigated (Aschersleben & Prinz, 1995; Bard et al., 1992). In recent years, oscillator models from dynamic systems theory, in which sensorimotor synchronization is understood as entrainment of rhythmic motor processes through the interaction with dynamic stimulus patterns, have been proven very useful in advancing our understanding of entrainment processes in rhythmic motor behavior (Large & Jones, 1999; Large & Palmer, 2002; McAuley & Jones, 2003; Clayton, Sager, & Will, 2005). Applied entrainment research has looked at intrinsic rhythmicity and frequency coupling in neural systems, for example, central pattern genera-tors for gait, rhythmically coordinated arm movements (Turvey, Schmidt, & Rosenblum, 1989), and other biological response systems (Kopell, 1990). Several studies have used auditory rhythm to entrain gait patterns in patients with stroke (Thaut, McIntosh, Prassas, & Rice, 1993; Thaut, McIntosh, & Rice, 1997) and Parkinson's disease (McIntosh, Thaut, & Rice, 1996) in clinically applied synchronization research (Thaut, Peterson, & McIntosh, 2005). However, as already indicated in the first chapter, despite a wealth of research dedicated to the topic, the specific neurophysi-ological processes that underlie time-coupling between rhythmic sensory input and motor output are poorly understood and only partly known. The present chapter first discusses some key issues in applying entrainment con-cepts to electrophysiological studies and then reports research investigating a core aspect of the underlying processes: the interaction between repetitive auditory stimuli and ongoing brain activity (brainwave oscillations), focus-ing on a range of stimulation rates (0.5 to 8Hz) that seems most relevant in human repetitive sensorimotor behavior, especially that involved in music making and perception.

Entrainment, Evoked Responses, and Induced Rhythms

A frequently neglected issue in entrainment research on brain activities is *whether the observed responses are a simple, passive consequence of the periodic stimuli producing a fixed neural response or whether they reflect active modification of ongoing brain activity by the stimulation.* As out-lined in Chapter 1, this distinction is crucial from a perspective of entrain-ment theory: Though both types of responses are synchronized with the stimuli, only the second case, involving more than one independent oscilla-tory process, would qualify as entrainment.

These two types of brain responses are often thought of in terms of evoked and induced responses, the latter term derived from Adrian's introduction of the term induced waves (Adrian, 1950) and Başar and Bullock's publication of *Induced Rhythms in the Brain* (Başar & Bullock, 1992). From an entrainment perspective, this practice is not unproblem-atic, and the problems lie with both notions. In Bullock's (1992) defini-tion, induced rhythms are oscillations caused or modified by stimuli or state changes that do not directly drive successive cycles. It seems, then, that entrained responses would form a subclass of induced responses: stimulus-induced modifications of ongoing oscillations. However, for Bullock, induced responses do not show rhythms presented in the stimuli, and he considers driven oscillations, oscillations that interact on a cycle-by-cycle basis, as a distinct category that can be subsumed under the category of evoked rhythms. Bullock himself, though, also seems to envisage an alternative, more convincing distinction when he writes, without any further comment:

> Başar et al. report examples of induced rhythms in the theta, alpha and gamma bands. They emphasize the working hypothesis that these evoked responses are stimulus-induced synchronization and enhancements of the spontaneous EEG. (Bullock, 1992, p. 14)

Although this statement might seem contradictory at first sight, it leads us right to the center of a longstanding controversy about the nature of event-related brain responses (ERPs). Though the study of ERPs is one of the methodological pillars of research on brain dynamics, there is no consensus on how event-locked brain activity occurs. Currently there are two alternative models. In the older view, the evoked activity that produces the ERPs is generated as fixed-polarity and fixed-latency neuronal activity superimposed on the background activity ofthe brain (see: Hillyard, 1985). Following the research of Sayers and colleagues (1974), a different interpretation developed (the oscillatory model) which suggests that ERPs are generated by reorganizing the phase spectra of ongoing brain activity. Though studies indicate that both types of responses, purely evoked as well as phase reorganization of ongoing activity, do occur, it is crucial for entrainment research to be able to distinguish between both of them. Theoretically, it is possible to make a distinction in terms of time-frequency analysis that is performed on single trials instead of averages: Superimposed fixed polarity evoked activity should produce changes in the power spectrum (measured as *event related spectral perturbation* or [ERSP]; Makeig, 1993), whereas stimulus-related phase reorganization of brain oscillations can be detected by changes stimuli produce in the inter-trial phase coherence (Makeig et al., 2002). (It is important that this analysis is performed on single trials because a pre-analysis averaging would eliminate or reduce responses, evoked as well as oscillatory, that are not strictly time-locked). However, Klimesch (1999) has pointed out that if evoked activity is strongly phase-locked to the stimulus, enhanced phase coherence measures could, in principle, be due to purely evoked responses. Consequently, if one finds simultaneous spectral power and phase coherence changes, it is impossible to decide whether this is due to only evoked activity or a joint evoked and oscillatory contribution to the ERP. Only a case of increased phase coherence without simultaneous changes in the power spectrum unambiguously indicates an underlying oscillatory process, as evoked responses always produce spectral power contributions.

If we make a distinction between purely evoked and induced responses on the basis of these operational criteria, then entrainment responses form a subclass of induced responses and they may also include (induced) responses that show rhythms present in the stimuli. On the other hand, evoked responses, even if time-locked and synchronized to the stimuli, would not qualify as entrainment responses as long as they produce only ERSPs, because they do not imply interacting oscillatory processes. (The foregoing discussion also clarifies that making the distinction between evoked and induced responses on the basis of the degree of time-locking is not a very useful criterion, because both can show a considerable range of variability in response latencies.)

Not all contributors to the present volume are going to subscribe to the definition of entrainment proposed here. In various disciplines entrainment is sometimes used synonymously with synchronization. However, as it has been demonstrated that synchronization can also occur between completely unrelated processes (Kreuz, 2003), it seems important to make a clear distinction between the identification of synchronization and the demonstration that synchronization is due to the interaction of active oscillatory processes, that is, the identification of entrainment. In the following presentation of some recent experimental studies it will be shown how this two-tier process actually works in practice and what the advantages of a clear distinction between synchronization and entrainment are for neurophysiological and neuropsychological studies.

EEG Waveforms

When we began analyzing the waveform of the brain responses to continuous stimulation, we found that for our repetition rates, ranging from 0.5 to 8Hz, the analyses were complicated by several factors. First, continuous stimulation produced waveforms different from those observed for intermittent single stimuli, pairs, or triplets. Second, there is a decrease in amplitude with increasing stimulation rates. Third, there is considerable ongoing activity, part of which does not seem to be independent of the experimental situation, as it is not effectively reduced by averaging. For stimulation rates higher than 4/s these factors make it difficult if not impossible to unambiguously identify the periodicity or individual peaks of the response waveform.

Most notably, the dominant N1 waves that characterize responses to discontinuous stimulation are strongly reduced, even at repetition rates as low as 0.5/s or 0.8/s. Instead, P2 and N2 are the largest response components for stimulation rates up to 3 or 4Hz (Figure 5.1). With increasing stimulation rates there is a reduction of peak amplitude throughout the range of rates applied in our experiments. Although this dependency seems to resemble the well-known reduction of the amplitude of the auditory evoked potential (AEP) for stimulus repetition rates faster than about 0.125Hz (for review: Näätänen & Picton, 1987), the changes that cause this reduction are different. Figure 5.1 shows a waveform rate series for one subject, each trace representing an average of 120, 1-sec epochs. For continuous stimulation, it is the P2–N2 peak-to-peak amplitude that decreases from ca.12μV at 0.5Hz to ca.3μV at a 4Hz stimulation rate. Our rate series indicates that amplitude reduction continues up to repetition rates of at least 8Hz and probably beyond. Similar observations have been reported in a stimulus-rate MEG study by Carver and colleagues (Carver et al. 2002).

In order to directly compare EEG responses to intermittent and continuous stimulation, we performed an experiment in which we used continuous stimulation as well as short stimulus sequences (a modification of the stimuli used by Fuentemilla, Marco-Pallars, & Grau, 2006). Subjects listened to four different stimuli:

1. 120 stimuli consisting of 4 tone sequences, with 1kHz tones of 75ms duration, 10 ms rise and fall time, 500 ms IOI, and an inter-sequence interval of 18.5 sec;
2. Same stimulus with 6 tones per sequence;

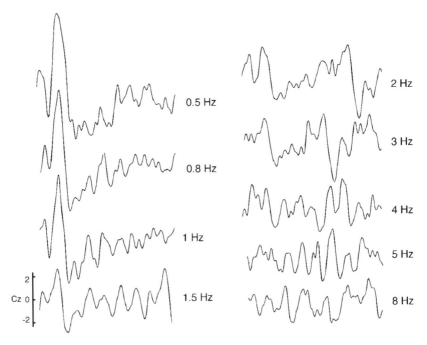

Figure 5.1   Rate series of EEG responses at the Cz electrode from one subject to 2 min acoustic stimulation by periodic drum sounds. Each trace is an average of 120, 1-sec epochs, stimulation rate is indicated to the right of each trace. Abscissa in ms, ordinate in μV, positive = up.

3. 2 min continuous stimulation with the same tones and 500 ms IOI;
4. 2 min continuous stimulation with sampled drum sounds with 500 ms IOI and the same peak amplitude as the tone stimuli.

The intermittent stimuli sequences yield basically the same results as in the Fuentemilla et al. (2006) study: The first stimulus in a sequence produces pronounced N1, P2, and P3 waves, the second stimulus produces reduced N1 and P2 waves with no noticeable P3. For subsequent stimuli (we tested up to 6) N1 reduced further but P2 as well as N2 showed slight increases (see trace A in Figure 5.2). In comparison, continuous stimulation produces waveforms with reduced N1 (smaller than any of the N1 responses in the intermittent condition) and marked P1, P2, and N2 responses (trace B and C in Figure 5.2).

EEG responses to intermittent and continuous stimulation clearly involve different brainwave components. The most conspicuous difference seems to be the absence of one or more N1 components, probably those that are related to the novelty aspects of the stimuli and related attentional processes

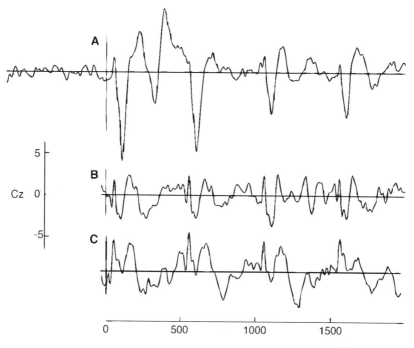

Figure 5.2 Comparison of waveforms following intermittent (A) and continuous (B, C) acoustic stimulation in one subject. Each trace is an average of 120 epochs. A: responses to 4-tone sequences (1kHz, 75 ms, 10 ms rise/fall time) with an inter-sequence interval of 18.5 sec. B: response to 2 min continuous stimulation with 1kHz tones (75 ms duration and 10 ms rise/fall time). C: response to 2 min continuous stimulation with sampled drum sounds; same peak amplitude as in B. For all traces stimulus onsets coincide with the time marks at 0, 500, 1000, and 1500 ms.

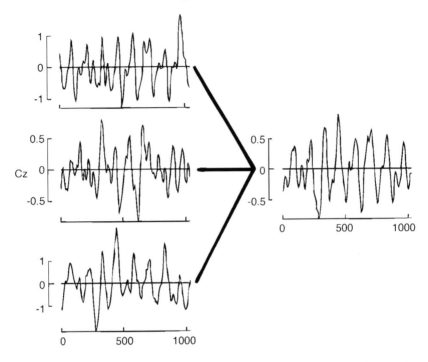

Figure 5.3 Averaged EEG responses at Cz to continuous 8Hz stimulation (drum sounds). On the left are averages (n = 160) from 3 different subjects; note partly opposite polarity across subjects at corresponding time points; on the right is the average for the 3 subjects; dots = stimulus onsets, abscissa in ms, ordinate μV, positive = up.

(for details see: Näätänen & Picton, 1987), and stronger background activity under continuous stimulation. However, as of the third response to the stimulus train, the intermittent stimulation produces a waveform (last two responses in trace A of Figure 5.2) that resembles that for continuous stimulation, especially in the region between P1 to N2.

At stimulation rates higher than 3Hz there is increasing overlap in the midlatency components. Additionally, with the reduced amplitude at these rates, the ongoing activity produces considerable variability of the responses, a factor that makes it difficult, if not impossible, to unequivocally identify peaks at rates higher than about 3 or 4Hz. The fact that averaging does not much reduce this variability indicates, as demonstrated by Arieli and colleagues (1996), that this ongoing activity is not independent from the stimulus situation. The superposition of the small-amplitude evoked activity and the related ongoing activity probably causes the stimulus periodicity to be obscured for stimulation rates from 4Hz to 8Hz (see Figure 5.1).

This ongoing activity contains clear subject-specific components, as illustrated in Figure 5.3. This figure shows averaged (160, 1-sec epochs each) waveforms in response to continuous 8Hz stimulation (drum sounds) for three subjects on the left. Despite the averages, there are non-vanishing differences between the subjects, with corresponding points in time sometimes having even opposite polarity, and at least for the middle trace, it would seem difficult to deduce the stimulus period from the waveform. Only the average over the subjects (trace on the right) brings out the time-locked periodicity, which still contains large-scale variations indicated by the amplitude fluctuations (despite the constant amplitude of the stimuli!) that have been suggested to be due to central habituation processes involving feedback loops (Spreng & Keidel, 1963; Spreng, 1975).

This brief analysis of EEG waveforms elicited in response to continuous acoustic stimulation clearly indicates that they are different from those produced in response to intermittent stimulation. For stimulation rates up to 4Hz, the most obvious difference is a reduced N1 wave, a relative prominence of P1 and P2, and a marked N2 for continuous stimulation. Peak-to-peak amplitude decreases with increasing stimulation rates, and at rates larger that 3Hz the stimulus periodicity becomes obscured, due to the relatively strong and not completely independent background activity. We therefore decided not to base our entrainment study on the analysis of the EEG waveform, but to perform a phase synchronization analysis using inter-trial coherence as a measure (Will & Berg, 2007).

Continuous Periodic Stimulation Experiment

We will now turn to the question of what brainwave synchronization phenomena can be observed under continuous periodic stimulation, and subsequently we will address the question of which of the synchronization phenomena can be understood as brainwave entrainment to external stimuli. As it turns out, periodic stimuli produce a variety of synchronization effects—all of which are potentially relevant to understand the effects of periodic sound stimuli like music—but only one of them meets the criteria of entrainment. In our main synchronization study (Will & Berg, 2007) we used Neher's (1961) stimulation paradigm in a slightly modified form. For acoustic stimuli we used digitally recorded drum sounds as well as clicks (0.005 s rectangular pulses) and pink noise (noise with an energy distribution matching human auditory frequency sensitivity). Recording periods with silence (no acoustic stimulation) and continuous pink noise served as controls and reference measures.

Subjects (N = 10; 5 female; mean age 26) were seated in an upright chair, wearing an EEG cap and listening to the stimuli via headphones with eyes closed. The peak SPL for the acoustic stimuli at the headphones was adjusted to 79 dB. Continuous EEG recordings were made while subjects listened to alternating 2-min periods of silence and randomly selected periodic stimuli or pink noise. The presentation sequence of repetition rates (from 1 to 8Hz in 1Hz steps) and control trials was counterbalanced across subjects. EEGs were recorded from 19 non-polarizable Ag/AgCl electrodes (impedance < 5 k) according to the international 1020 system, referenced against common linked earlobes. Sampling rate was 256Hz with a time constant of 0.3 s (upper frequency limit = 70Hz). Phase synchronization analysis was performed on registrations from the vertex electrode (Cz), which yielded the largest response.

To analyze the synchronization between stimuli and brainwaves, we used the stimulus-locked inter-trial coherence (ITC), applied to 3-sec epochs of the EEG recordings. The ITC is the average (over trials) of the spectral estimate of the (amplitude-) normalized power spectrum and describes the phase alignment or correlation (coherence) across trials, independent of amplitude variations. As each trial is time-locked to the stimulus sequence, the ITC is also a measure of synchronization between stimulus and brain response. ITC calculations were done with a MATLAB-script based on the phasecoher function from EEGLAB (Delorme & Makeig, 2004). We calculated the

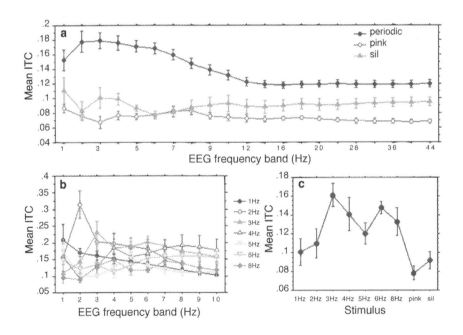

Figure 5.4 Grand average (n = 10) of meanITC. A: MeanITC for silent condition (sil), continuous pink noise stimulation (pink) and the mean for all periodic stimulations (periodic) for all analyzed EEG frequency bands. B: MeanITC responses for 1–8Hz repetition rates in the delta, theta, and alpha range. C: MeanITC in the lower gamma range (20Hz). Error bars = ±1 S. E.

spectral estimate with a 3-cycles tapered wavelet for 1Hz frequency bands from 1 to 10Hz, 2Hz bands from 12 to 22Hz and 4Hz bands from 26 to 44Hz. Because of the window effects, only ITC values from the middle 1-sec epoch were considered in the following. Averaging over these 1-sec epochs, we obtained the meanITC for each stimulus condition and subject. As our experimental paradigm does not allow for determination of a significance

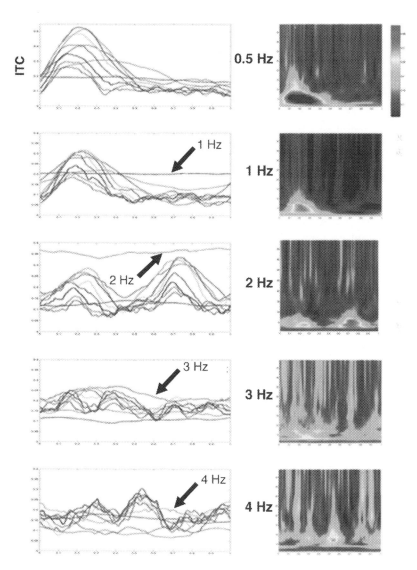

Figure 5.5 Grand average (n = 10) for ITCs for EEG frequency bands 1–10Hz during 1 sec EEG epochs for stimulus rates from 0.5 to 4Hz. Left column: time/ITC plots, right column: time/frequency band (1–44Hz) with ITC as color code.

level of the ITC through comparison with a pre-stimulus baseline, we tested the significance in an analysis of variance of ITC values for the three experimental conditions (non-stimulation, noise, periodic stimulation).

Analysis of variance (ANOVA) performed on the grand average (all subjects, n = 10) showed a significant effect of stimulus condition (periodic stimuli, noise, silence), but no significant effects for EEG frequency bands; there was also no interaction between these two factors (condition: $F[2, 9] = 79.06$, $p < 0.001$; frequency band: $F[20, 9] = 0.39$, $p = 0.9618$). The main effect for condition was due to the increased phase coherence under periodic stimulation (see: Figure 6.4), whereas pink noise slightly reduces phase coherence in the range above the alpha waves (8–12Hz). A post-hoc test did not show any significant coherence differences between the effects of periodic drum and click stimuli ($F[1, 9] = 0.112$, $p > 0.7$). The meanITC indicates that the synchronization responses in the beta and gamma range (13–44Hz) consist of a more or less constant increase in coherence over this entire range, whereas the response in the delta to alpha range (1–12Hz) is larger, varies with the EEG frequency bands, and shows a maximum at around 3Hz. A similar distribution of synchronization strength is found when the mean ITC is analyzed with respect to stimulation rates (Figures 5.4b, 5.4c). In the beta and gamma range, response curves are flat or have a shallow slope for all stimulation rates and show response maxima for 3 and 6Hz repetition rates. In contrast, responses in the delta, theta, and alpha range show a marked frequency dependency, with stimulation rates from 1 to 5Hz producing maxima in the respective EEG frequency bands and 2Hz stimulations generating the largest responses.

Figure 5.4b also suggests that the responses in the delta and theta range may be composite responses, consisting of frequency-band-specific components centered in the delta range and non-specific components with maxima in the theta band. Responses up to 5Hz repetition rates each have a

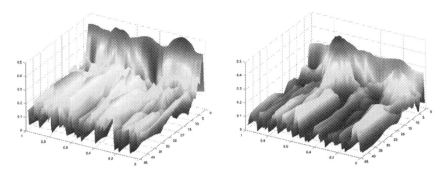

Figure 5.6   Average ITC distribution during 1-s epochs and across EEG bands (1–44Hz) for two subjects. Both were exposed to 2 min of acoustic stimulation with identical (!) sampled drum sounds presented at a rate of 2/s. x-axis = time (sec), y-axis = ITC, z-axis = EEG frequency bands.

maximum in the corresponding frequency bands, with 2Hz producing considerably larger values than the other rates (for 1, 2, and 3Hz the maxima are absolute, for 4 and 5Hz relative). Stimulation rates of 6 and 8Hz do not produce response peaks at the corresponding EEG frequency band but show relative maxima at the subharmonics of 3 and 4Hz, respectively. All stimulation rates produce a second, broader response peak (only a raised level for 2Hz stimuli) in the theta/alpha range.

Analysis of the actual time course of the ITC supports the idea of a composite response in the delta and theta range (Figure 5.5): The frequency-specific peaks in the meanITC responses are produced by a tonic ITC component in the frequency band corresponding to the stimulation rate (marked by arrows in Figure 5.5). This component has a pronounced maximum around the 2Hz stimulation rate, falling off sharply with lower and higher rates. The second component is a phasic ITC response in all frequency bands above the band corresponding to the stimulation rate. The peak amplitude decreases with the repetition rate, though there is a relative maximum for 2Hz stimuli. The stimulus periodicity that is reflected in this

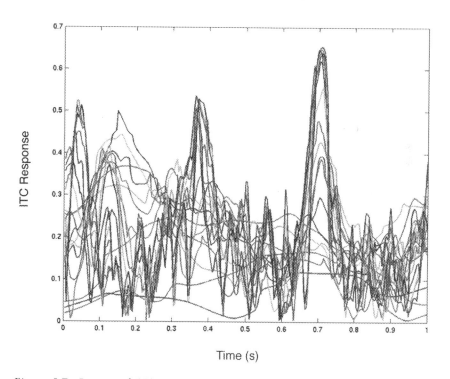

Time (s)

Figure 5.7 Pattern of ITC responses in the 1–44Hz bands for one subject. The graph shows the ITC responses (ordinate) averaged over 120, 1-sec epochs (abscissa). Stimulus rate was 3Hz. In this subject the beta/gamma band response (dense set of curves, all with a similar modulation of ca.20Hz) was unusually strong in comparison with the delta/theta/alpha band response.

component up to a rate of 2Hz gets obscured at higher rates because the ITC response peaks do not appear to be sharply time-locked and show considerable inter-subject variability (Figure 5.6).

Notably, though all stimulus sounds had fixed and constant amplitudes, those peaks of the phasic ITC responses that reflect stimulus periodicities do not attain a constant height for subsequent stimuli. In some subjects, though not in all, this leads to a clear grouping of the ITC response. The strength of the grouping, as well as the grouping pattern, was found to vary across subjects; however, there seem to be some dominant patterns, as indicated by Figure 5.5 where the 2Hz stimulation produces a clear pattern of 1 sec length, even though the figure shows an average over all 10 subjects. Figure 5.6 shows two individual responses, one relatively symmetric, the other strongly asymmetric. These findings suggest that the phase synchronization response is patterned or modulated by stimulus-independent factors, and one possible explanation may be that they reflect subjective grouping of the stimulus sequence by the subjects.

A third component is the synchronization response in the 14–44Hz EEG bands (Figure 5.7). It seems to consist of two subcomponents, an ITC modulation by delta and lower theta frequencies (corresponding to the stimulus periodicities), and an increased 20–26Hz ITC modulation. These subcomponents have not been identified in studies using short stimulus sequences and may be characteristic for longer stimulation periods (Will & Berg, 2007).

Continuous Stimulation and Entrainment

Having shown that continuous periodic auditory stimulation leads to a significant increase in stimulus-locked brainwave synchronization, the interesting question is now whether this synchronization is due to entrainment or not. In other words, is the increased coherence due to changes in ongoing brain activities or is it just a consequence of the fact that each auditory stimulus evokes a neural response of a certain latency and frequency content? Is the increased synchronization due to evoked or induced (see above) activity? And, if it is induced, is it of an oscillatory nature?

1. The delta and lower theta range show a marked stimulus rate dependent increase in ITC, with 2Hz stimulations generating the largest responses (in the 2Hz EEG band meanITC for 2Hz stimulation rates is about double that for 1 or 3Hz). The existence of a response maximum is clearly incompatible with the idea that increased ITC is a mere reflection of stimulus sequence. Furthermore, this response is tonic and, as such, does not reflect the periodicity of the stimulus sequence. *We therefore argue that this response reflects the reorganization (i.e., stimulus-related phase synchronization) of ongoing activity and describe it as delta wave entrainment to periodic external acoustic stimulation.* Interestingly, the maximum of the tonic ITC response is found at a stimulation rate close to the suggested optimal

tempo (between ca. 1.5 and 2.5Hz) of human repetitive perceptuo-motor behavior (e.g. preferred tempo in listening to and making of music, accuracy in detecting deviant event interval durations, tapping synchronization, etc.; see: Van Noorden & Moelants, 1999).

We have recently started an experiment to determine the location of the maximum response with a better resolution. Surprisingly, preliminary results from 4 subjects (Figure 5.8) seem to indicate that there might be two maxima, one between 1.8 and 2Hz, the other between 2.2 and 2.3Hz, separated by a marked drop in meanITC at 2.1Hz. At present the significance of this double peak structure, whether it might, for example, indicate the differential involvement of different processes, is not clear. With the findings of Carver et al. (2002) it seems possible that this gap is connected with the transition towards a steady state response that starts around 2 Hz. In any case, the correspondence between stimulation rates for maximum ITC responses and the range of optimal tempi identified in other studies strongly suggests a connection between the two: neural mechanisms leading to the tonic synchronization response peaks may also be involved in determining the preferred tempo.

2. A second ITC component was identified as a phasic response in all frequency bands of the theta and alpha range above the band corresponding to the stimulation rate. The fact that it is a phasic response and that its peak amplitude decreases with the repetition rate might be seen as an indication that this component mainly reflects the coherence of stimulus evoked activity.

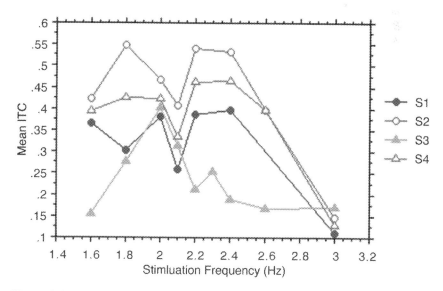

Figure 5.8 MeanITC responses from four subjects listening to 2 min segments of periodic drum stimuli with repetition rates between 1.6 and 3Hz. Responses recorded at Cz with linked earlobe references.

Unfortunately, our continuous stimulation paradigm does not permit us to directly test whether the increased ITC is accompanied by an increase in ERSP or not (if we were to compare the ERSP for the periodic stimulation periods with the ERSP for the control periods, e.g. silence, it could be argued that these two conditions relate to different brain states and, therefore, their comparison is not conclusive). However, our modification of the Fuentemilla et al. (2006) experiment suggests a different interpretation. In that experiment we used periodic stimulus sequences with 4 to 6 tones (1kHz, 75 ms, 10 ms rise/fall time, constant amplitude) or sampled drum sounds, repeatedly presented with an inter-sequence interval of 18.5 s, and we obtained similar results as Fuentemilla et al. (2006) when analyzing the ERSP and ITC of these responses (Figure 5.9).

In our experiment, only the responses to the first and, though much less, the second stimulus within a sequence showed a significant increase in spectral power, combined with a significant increase in ITC. All subsequent stimuli in a sequence only show a significant ITC increase. This suggests that for periodic sequences and, ultimately, continuous stimulation, only the

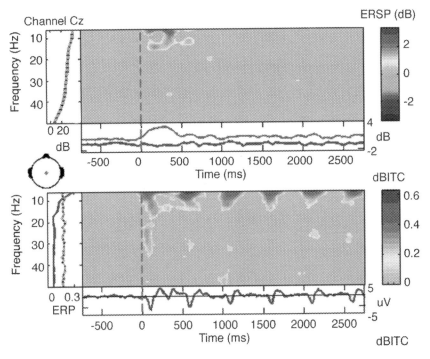

Figure 5.9 Comparison of event-related spectral perturbation (ERSP) and inter-trial coherence (ITC) for intermittent acoustic stimulation with 6-tone sequences (1kHz, 75 ms, 10 ms rise/fall time, inter-sequence interval = 18.5 sec). Analysis is done on 480, 4-sec epochs, 120 from each of 4 subjects. Electrode location = Cz with linked earlobe references.

first or first two stimuli produce significant ERSP as well as ITC responses, and, as explained above, it can not be decided whether responses to these stimuli are purely evoked or a combination of evoked and phase resetting responses. However, responses to the third and later stimuli are not produced by changes in spectral power distribution but by a phase resetting mechanism, that is, they reflect reorganization of ongoing activity.

With these results it seems justified to assume that the phasic ITC response in the case of continuous stimulation is not accompanied by an ERSP response and can, therefore, be classified as an induced response: Periodic stimulation causes a stimulus-locked phase-resetting over a broad frequency range (above the stimulation frequency), but the phase adjustments dissipate immediately without causing entrainment. Although the phasic response can be understood as an induced response it is not, at the same time, an entrainment response.

3. The increased coherence throughout the EEG frequency bands from 13–44Hz shows an absolute maximum for 3Hz and a second, smaller maximum for 6Hz stimulus rates (see Figure 5.4c). A posthoc analysis indicates that meanITC for 3 and 6Hz in the 20Hz EEG band are significantly different from the silent and pink conditions (Bonferroni-Dunn $p < 0.0001$) as well as from the 1Hz stimulation (Bonferroni-Dunn $p < 0.0001$), whereas the meanITCs for the 1 and 2Hz stimulation are not different from the control conditions (Will & Berg, 2007). This third synchronization response appears to contain two subcomponents, an ITC modulation in the delta and lower theta range corresponding to the stimulus periodicity and an increased 20–26Hz ITC modulation. The 20–26Hz modulation is most likely an induced response (not related to stimulus features and/or determined by stimulus rates), but the status of the modulation in the delta and lower theta range is unclear. It is possible that this modulation is another case of cross-frequency interactions that have been demonstrated in a number of species and brain regions, and, as such, it might be involved in integration of several neural networks or might be utilized for phase coding (Jensen & Colgin, 2007).

It seems that these subcomponents do not show up in studies using short stimulus sequences. Neither Fuentemilla et al. (2006) nor our own study on short stimuli sequences (see Figure 5.9) show any consistent and significant ERSP or ITC responses in the 20–49Hz frequency range. These different results could be due to the slightly different analytical methods (for intermittent stimulation ITC significance is calculated in reference to a 1000 ms pre-stimulus baseline) or, more likely, the different experimental design. As augmented synchronization in the 14–44Hz EEG bands is probably mediated by increased activity in the 20–26Hz range, it is possible that this is either not present in short stimulus sequences or rises to significance only under prolonged stimulation. However this may be, indications are that this synchronization response in the beta/gamma range is most likely not an entrainment response to the stimuli: Although 3Hz stimulation produces the largest response, the response shows a nearly constant strength throughout the beta/gamma range and therefore is not frequency specific.

CONCLUSIONS

The studies presented above demonstrate that periodic acoustic stimuli have specific effects on the activity of the brain that are different from intermittent or single stimuli. For continuous periodic stimulation, the novelty effect disappears with the second or third stimulus, as indicated by the reduction of the N1 component, and the brain continues to respond with adjustment of the brainwave phase, that is, synchronization in various frequency bands but no changes in spectral energy (as measured by the ERSP). Only one of the synchronization phenomena described above, the tonic increase in ITC in the delta wave band, meets the criteria for entrainment. *Interestingly, the maximum of this response is found at a stimulation rate of about 2Hz, which corresponds to the preferred tempo determined by other studies (e.g., Van Noorden & Moelants, 1999), and we suggest that this tonic response might constitute an important component linking sensory and motor domains in music perception and production.* The other synchronization phenomena described here do not seem to meet entrainment criteria:

1. These responses are not frequency-specific in the sense that they show nearly constant synchronization strength of over a wide range of brainwave frequencies.
2. The phasic response is an intermittent synchronization that quickly dissipates and then reappears following each incoming stimulus and thus does not lead to entrainment.

In no way does this imply that these (non-entrainment) synchronization phenomena are not relevant for the effects of music on the human mind and body—quite to the contrary. The point is much more that the above results indicate that periodic acoustic stimuli (e.g., music) produce a variety of synchronization responses, not all of which are entrainment responses; in other words, not every brain response to periodic stimuli necessarily involves entrainment.

Therefore, a clear distinction between the different synchronization phenomena is important in order to arrive at an adequate interpretation and understanding of the effects that periodic acoustic stimulation, like music, can have on the functioning of the brain. On the other hand, there is evidence that the observed synchronization in the beta and gamma bands is an important element to explain the reported effects of music on learning (Thaut et al., 1997) and the cross-frequency interaction between delta/lower theta and gamma bands may contribute to improved memory processes similar to the theta and gamma band interaction in the Lisman and Idiart model (1995).

It is interesting to note that, besides subject-specific variability in latency and amplitude, the synchronization responses show grouping patterns in several subjects. Despite the fact that all stimuli in a sequence have exactly the same physical features (amplitude, duration, rise and fall times) these subjects show a grouping of the ITC response spanning two or more stimuli (see Figure 5.6 for a pattern covering two stimuli). Obviously, synchronization is not just established as an automatic response of brainwaves to external stimulation, but it is influenced by internal states and ongoing cognitive processes of the subjects. It is possible, for example, that the observed ITC patterns are a reflection of the subjects' perceptual grouping; this can only be demonstrated, however, in further experimental studies.

The studies reported here are only concerned with the effects of one main experimental variable, stimulation rate, or in musical terms, that of musical tempo. Other musical variables like timbre, melody, or rhythm, have not been considered, although they might have a considerable effect on the tuning in to a specific music. This does not diminish the significance of the above results; it just says that in actual performances many more processes are going on that may have an influence on the state of mind of the participant or performer. Even if we stick with our main variable, than it is also obvious that the exposure to continuous stimulation for 2 to 4 minutes in no way represents stimulation periods typically found in, for example, ceremonial performances, and there are indications that long-term exposure (> 5 minutes) leads to additional changes in brain activity,[2] *suggesting that the synchronization responses identified above may not be invariant under long-term stimulus exposure.*

NOTES

1. For reprints, see: sccn.ucsd.edu/~scott
2. See Jovanov & Maxfield, Chapter 2 of this volume.

REFERENCES

Adrian, E. D. (1950). The electrical activity of the mammalian olfactory bulb. *Electroencephalography and Clinical Neurophysiology, 2*, 377–387.

Arieli, A., Sterkin, A., Grinvald, A., & Aertsen, A. (1996). Dynamics of ongoing activity: Explanation of large variability in evoked cortical responses. *Science, 273*, 1868–1871.

Aschersleben, G., & Prinz, W. (1995). Synchronizing actions with events: The role of sensory information. *Perception and Psychophysics, 57*, 305–317.

Bard, C., Paillard, J., Lajoie, Y., Fleury, M., Teasdale, N., Forget, R., & Lamarre, Y. (1992). Role of afferent information in the timing of motor commands: A comparative study with a deafferented patient. *Neuropsychologia, 30*, 201–206.

Başar, E., & Bullock, T. H. (Eds.). (1992). *Induced rhythms in the brain.* Boston, Basel, Berlin: Birckhuser.

Bullock, T. H. (1992). Introduction to induced rhythms: A widespread, heterogeneous class of oscillations. In E. Başar & T. H. Bullock (Eds.), *Induced rhythms in the brain* (pp. 1–26). Boston, Basel, Berlin: Birckhuser.

Carver, F. W., Fuchs, A., Jantzen, K. J., Kelso, J. A. S. (2002). Spatiotemporal analysis of the neuromagnetic response to rhythmic auditory stimulation: rate dependence and transient to steady-state transition. *Clinical Neurophysiology, 113*, 1921–1931.

Clayton, M., Sager, R., & Will, U. (2005). In time with the music: The concept of entrainment and its significance for ethnomusicology. *ESEM-Counterpoint, No. 1, European Meetings in Ethnomusicology, Vol. 11.*

Cohn, R. (1952). A visual analysis and a study of latency of the photically driven EEG. *Electroencephalography and Clinical Neurophysiology, 4*, 297–301.

Delorme, A., & Makeig, S. (2004). EEGLAB: An open source toolbox for analysis of single-trial EEG dynamics. *Journal of Neuroscience Methods, 134*, 9–21.

Dobie, R. A. (2001). *Medical-legal evaluation of hearing loss* (2nd ed.). San Diego, CA: Singular.

Durand, V. M., & Barlow, D. H. (2006). *Essentials of abnormal psychology* (4th ed.). Boston: Wadsworth.

Fuentemilla, L., Marco-Pallars, J., & Grau, C. (2006). Modulation of spectral power and of phase resetting of EEG contributes differentially to the generation of auditory event related potentials. *NeuroImage, 30*, 909–916.

Gazzaniga, M. S. (Ed.). (2000). *The new cognitive neurosciences* (2nd ed.). Cambridge, MA: MIT.

Hillyard, S. A. (1985). Electrophysiology of human selective attention. *Trends In Neurosciences, 8*, 400–405.

Jensen, O., & Colgin, L. L. (2007). Cross-frequency coupling between neuronal oscillators. *Trends in Cognitive Sciences, 11*(7), 267–269.

Klimesch, W. (1999). EEG alpha and theta oscillations reflect cognitive and memory performance: A review and analysis. *Brain Research Reviews, 29*, 169–195.

Kopell, N. (1990). Toward a theory of modeling central pattern generators. In A. H. Cohen, S. Rossignol, & S. Grillner (Eds.), *Neural control of rhythmic movements in vertebrates* (pp. 369–413). New York: Wiley.

Kreuz, T. (2003) Measuring Synchronization in Model Systems and Electrocephalographic Time Series from Epilepsy Patients. NCI Series Vol. 21, Jülich: Jogn von Neumann Institute for Computing.

Large, E. W., & Jones, M. R. (1999). The dynamics of attending: How people track time-varying events. *Psychological Review, 106*, 119–159.

Large, E. W., & Palmer, C. (2002). Perceiving temporal regularity in music. *Cognitive Science, 26*, 1–37.

Lisman, J. E., & Idiart, M. A. (1995). Storage of 7+/-2 short-term memories in oscillatory subcycles. *Science, 267*, 1512–1515.

Makeig, S. (1993). Auditory event-related dynamics of the EEG spectrum and effects of exposure to tones. *Electroencephalography and Clinical Neurophysiology, 86*, 283–293.

Makeig, S., Jung, T. P., Bell, A. J., Ghahremani, D., & Sejnowski, T. J. (1997). Blind separation of auditory event related brain responses into independent components. *Proceedings of the National Academy of Sciences USA, 94*, 10979–10984.

Makeig, S., Westerfield, M., Bell, Jung, T. P., Enghoff, S., Townsend, J., . . . Sejnowski, T. J. (2002). Dynamic brain sources of visual evoked responses. *Science*, *295*, 690–694.

McAuley, J. D., & Jones, M. R. (2003). Modeling effects of rhythmic context on perceived duration: A comparison of interval and entrainment approaches to short-interval timing. *Journal of Experimental Psychology: Human Perception and Performance*, *29*, 1102–1125.

McIntosh, G. C., Thaut, M. H., & Rice, R. R. (1996). Rhythmic Auditory Stimulation (RAS) as entrainment and therapy technique in gait of stroke and Parkinson's disease patients. *MusicMedicine*, *2*, 145–152.

Näätänen, R., & Picton, T. (1987). The N1 wave of the human electric and magnetic response to sound: A review and an analysis of the component structure. *Psychphysiology*, *24*(4), 375–425.

Neher, A. (1961). Auditory driving observed with scalp electrodes in normal subjects. *Electroencephalography and Clinical Neurophysiology*, *13*, 449–451.

Persinger, M. A. (1987). *Neuropsychological bases of god beliefs*. New York: Praeger.

Sayers, B. M., Beagley, H. A., & Hensall, W. R. (1974). The mechanism of auditory evoked EEG responses. *Nature*, *247*, 481–483.

Spreng, M. (1975). Langsame Rindenpotentiale, objektive Audiometrie und Psychoakustik. In W. D. Keidel (Ed.), *Physiologie des Gehrs. Akustische Informationsverarbeitung* (pp. 277–358). Stuttgart : Georg Thieme.

Spreng, M., & Keidel, W. D. (1963). Human evoked cortical responses to auditory stimuli: Interaction, time course of adaptation, influence of stimuli parameters. In J. W. Duyff (Ed.), *Abstracts XXIInd International Congress of Physiological Sciences, Leyden. International Congress Series 48* (p. 1010). Excerta Medica Foundation, Amsterdam, 1962.

Stetson, R. H. (1905). A motor theory of rhythm and discrete succession. *Psychological Review 12*, 250–270 (Part I), 293–350 (Part II).

Stevens, L. T. (1886). On the time sense. *Mind*, *11*, 393–404.

Thaut, M. H., McIntosh, G. C., Prassas, S. G., & Rice, R. R. (1993). Effect of rhythmic cuing on temporal stride parameters and EMG patterns in hemiparetic stroke patients. *Journal of Neurologic Rehabilitation*, *7*, 1993, 9–16.

Thaut, M. H., McIntosh, G. C., & Rice, R. R. (1997). Rhythmic facilitation of gait training in hemiparetic stroke rehabilitation. *Journal of Neurological Sciences*, *151*, 207–212.

Thaut, M. H., Peterson, D. A., & McIntosh, G. C. (2005). Temporal entrainment of cognitive functions. Musical mnemonics induce brain plasticity and oscillatory synchrony in neural networks underlying memory. *Annals of the New York Academy of Sciences*, *1060*, 243–254.

Turvey, M. T., Schmidt, R. C., & Rosenblum, L. D. (1989). Clock and motor components in absolute coordination of rhythmic movements. *Neuroscience*, *33*, 1–10.

Van Noorden, L. & Moelants, D. (1999). Resonance in the perception of musical pulse. *Journal of New Music Research*, *28*(I), 43–66.

Wallin, N. L. (1991). *Biomusicology*. Stuyvesant, NY: Pendragon.

Walter, V. J., & Walter, W. G. (1949). The central effects of rhythmic sensory stimulation. *Electroencephalography and Clinical Neurophysiology*, *1*, 57–86.

Will, U., & Berg, E. (2007). Brainwave synchronization and entrainment to periodic stimuli. *Neuroscience Letters*, *424*, 55–60.

Part II

Clinical Implications of Rhythmic Entrainment Research

6 Using Rhythmic Auditory Stimulation for Rehabilitation

Concetta M. Tomaino

PREFACE

Rhythmic music has a wide range of clinical applications for the rehabilitation of people with neurological impairments. The past 10 years have brought a surge of psychological and neuroscientific research relevant to the neuro-psycho-physical functioning of many different patient populations. Much of this work has informed the practice of music therapy, particularly the branches of music therapy that rely heavy on rhythmic cueing and entrainment. This review will highlight the state of current research and interventions, and suggest future developments necessary to continue the growth of this field.

INTRODUCTION TO MUSIC THERAPY

For the past 30 years I have observed and studied the effects of music therapy in a variety of patient populations, and it became clear to me, very early on, that there is something particular about music that allows for the stimulation of residual cognitive functioning. One of my first clinical experiences was on the dementia unit of a small nursing home where patients with Alzheimer's disease, multi-infarct dementia and/or vascular dementia were treated. When I arrived there, the medical staff told me that I should not expect any responses from these patients due to the severity of their impaired mental states—some were totally withdrawn and non-responsive, others extremely agitated. Nevertheless, the staff considered the possibility that music might be helpful, that it might provide a momentary respite for these otherwise lost individuals.

As I settled in that day, I began singing to them. Those who were reportedly unresponsive opened their eyes and looked in my direction. Those who were agitated calmed down. Many of them began to sing the words along with me. It was evident that despite cognitive impairments, these patients still possessed the capability for mental processing. From that moment I began to question what it is about music that could allow for such responses in those deemed to be unresponsive. I wanted to know how it was possible that individuals who where so cognitively impaired, by medical standards, could understand what I was doing. And most significantly, I knew it was crucial to learn more about the aspects music that let these patients actively engage and meaningfully interact with other people—something rarely possible for someone with advanced Alzheimer's disease.

Thirty years ago there was no scientific explanation for how music could stimulate such functioning in people who seemed so functionless. With the growth in the field of music therapy and the advancement of neuroscience in the area of music cognition, many of these clinical observations can now be explained.

Current clinical research indicates that music and the components of music, that is, rhythm, melody, harmony, can stimulate complex cognitive, affective, and sensorimotor processes in the brain, processes whose functions can be generalized and transferred to non-musical, therapeutic ends (Cohen, 1988, 1992; Tomaino, 1993; Repp, 2001, 2002). This is possible because music is processed in many areas of the brain. Research in music perception indicates that pitch is processed in the right temporal lobes, the same area that governs speech prosody (Patel, Peretz, Tramo, & Raymonde, 1998; Patel & Balaban, 2001). Memory systems can be stimulated by the associative memories connected to a particular piece of music or the harmonic structures that induce emotional responses (Tomaino, 1993). The processing of rhythmic cues (rhythm being a time-ordered or temporal process) involves the prefrontal motor cortex, the cerebellum, and other areas resulting in the stimulation of various neural networks. *The result of the complex interaction of music with areas distributed throughout the brain is that it has the ability to engage patients with disabilities who have difficulties in executive functioning, to bypass their functional and psychological impairments, and effect therapeutic outcomes.*

Music therapy is appropriate for most patients, regardless of their functional and cognitive abilities, because music can provoke responses from conscious and subconscious levels of awareness. Some of the most extensively researched and practiced music therapy techniques include rhythmic auditory stimulation and sensory enhancement using musical patterns for limb movement and gait training, musically cued speech for persons with non-fluent aphasia (impairment in producing meaningful words, phrases, and sentences), and relaxation training

with rhythmic auditory stimulation at slow tempos. For the purposes of this chapter, the term *music therapy* principally refers to active music therapy, that is, the interaction between the therapist and the client, in which the music therapist manipulates music/sound/rhythm in real-time to maximize the therapeutic benefit. The discussion will focus on interventions that rely on rhythm as their primary therapeutic component. Situations that involve the passive use of music will be indicated.[1]

RHYTHMIC MUSIC AND MOTOR MOVEMENT

In recent years, an increased interest in research on enriched environments, patterned sensory stimulation, and neural plasticity has blossomed. Patterned sensory activity is important to human development because it influences the organization and development of cortical circuits (Gao & Pallas, 1999; also see Chapters 8 and 9). Music therapists have become interested in this line of research, reasoning that if patterned auditory signaling enhances neural development, then the importance of rhythm in early developmental processes in children, as well as recovery from nerve injury in adults, may be of crucial therapeutic value. Moreover, clinicians want to investigate the extent to which enriched sensory stimuli can excite and reengage and/or form new connections to bypass damaged neural networks. Recent research supports this type of treatment approach.

Auditory processing occurs at various levels, with auditory tracts intersecting other sensory tracts throughout the brain from brainstem to cortex. Because of this arrangement, and, in part, because of the body's overall sensitivity to repetitive rhythms in the environment (Namerow et al., 1974; Condon, 1975; Haas, Distenfeld, & Axen, 1986; Thaut, McIntosh, Prassas, & Rice, 1992; Isaichev, Derevyankin, Koptelov, & Sokolov, 2001), rhythmic auditory stimulation seems to be able to entrain intrinsic rhythms in lower brain regions, and in the process, excite higher sensory tracts (Thaut, Miller, & Schauer, 1998; Large, Fink, & Kelso, 2002).

For example, we know that certain rhythmic patterns can drive or excite the motor cortex to coordinate movement. Studies by Thaut et al. (1998) and Large and colleagues (2002) indicate that auditory rhythm provides very precise temporal ordered information to the brain, which the motor system can access. This access can occur at a subconscious level making auditory rhythm a powerful tool for those who have lost executive functioning, that is, the ability to plan motor tasks on their own. This research complements findings that natural and spontaneous body movements can be an outward representation of internal timing mechanisms. For example, brain imaging studies show that there is an increase in activity in the prefrontal motor cortex in precise intervals in anticipation of a sequenced motor activity such as finger tapping at 1 sec intervals (Vafaee & Gjedde, 2004; Kudo et al., 2004).

In many of our patients with neurological diseases, initiation is a key problem. They often tell us that they feel like they want to move, but that they can't do it on their own. Interestingly, we may observe that this movement is possible spontaneously or in another context. In some cases, the difficulty lies in the fact the patient must think through the movements involved in specific tasks, rather than responding automatically. This type of decision/initiation related thinking is referred to as executive functioning—it is often damaged in those with traumatic brain injuries. Despite these difficulties, we've found that in many cases, patients may be coaxed into functioning through spontaneous activity with the right stimulus.

Rhythm, then, can be used to entrain movement when independent movement, initiation, or balance is a problem. With diseases like Parkinson's or stroke, where the internal initiation or sequential patterning of movement may be damaged, cueing of specific patterns through an outside source can allow for such functioning to be initiated (McIntosh, Thaut, Rice, Brown, & Prassas, 1997). Rhythm, as a time-ordered auditory cue, can help improve walking in those with other types of gait problems as well (Straum, 1983; Liberzon & Brown, 1998; Tomaino, 1998b; Howe, Lovgreen, Cody, Ashton, & Oldham, 2003). In these individuals, rhythmic music helps them initiate movement when they get frozen, helps coordinate the evenness of how they move, or becomes a template for organizing a series of movements. However, this process is not automatic. For a rhythmic cue to be useful therapeutically, it must entrain motor function on a subconscious level[2] while stimulating a conscious impulse or will to move in the patient. The music therapist explores various rhythmic patterns or musical styles with the patient to establish which patterns will help with walking, balance, and other motions. In these patients, the use of rhythm as an auditory cue to help structure time and stimulate the synchronization of physical functioning is often extremely effective. By attending to the auditory cue, rather than thinking about how to move, such individuals find that initiation, balance, coordination, and the performance of consecutive tasks are enhanced. Providing rhythm to supplement a sense of movement through the modulation of tempi enables the person to follow rather than initiate. The slight change in orientation, that is, following rather than initiating, enables for the improved functioning to be attained.

A casual observer might assume that these patients have lost a crucial skill (independent movement, balance, etc.), however, these patients may actually only have lost the ability to access that skill. We often think of memory as being related to history or facts names, places, dates, etc. But skills are also memories, memories of how to do things, like riding a bike, dancing, eating, or walking. Many patients that have lost this type of functioning may appear, and may be, depressed, lethargic, rigid, unmotivated— but often their primary issue is not psychological, but neurological. Actions that are rhythmic in nature can be stimulated or reinforced through rhythmic signals, ie rhythmic cueing. Through the appropriate use of music, residual functioning can be stimulated, and the psychological symptoms or effects of a previous lack of functioning can be eased and reduced.

For example, a patient of mine with a weakness on one side due to a stroke, would drag his left leg when walking with a cane. We found that when he walked with rhythmic music, he would lift his left leg and step exactly in time with the music without dragging his leg at all. He told us that when he walked to music he thought of dancing, and so his steps were different. The key difference here was that although he was still walking, his movement was now initiated and influenced by the music, rather than his self-initiated impulse to walk which had been impaired.

Some of my patients with Parkinson's disease (PD), for example, respond very well to a basic metronomic beat that cues, and is in synchrony with, their gait.[3] However, there are others for whom the accent has to be on the upbeat (falls between their steps) as in some Latin, jazz, and Irish dance rhythms. The upbeat pulse, they remark, gives them a lift to free their movement. Obviously, the stimuli and perceptual processes at work here differ, nevertheless, the therapeutic impact on initiation and improved gait are similar. In a clinical example I use often (filmed in 2006) a woman with bradykinesia (very slow movement) is reaching out to her aid to assist her to walk along a corridor. The music therapist, who is also in the corridor, begins to play "New York, New York" on a portable keyboard in an upbeat swing tempo. The patient, who has PD and starts off very slowly, shuffling down the hall, quickly entrains her gait to the rhythm, one hand holding her aid, the other loosely swaying to the music. By the time she gets to the end of the corridor (approximately 30 feet) she lets go of her aid's hand, turns around on her own, and walks back towards the therapist, swinging both arms and walking upright, in perfect tempo to the rhythmic cues of the music. This effect lasts as long as the music lasts. Unlike a medication that takes time to kick in, this effect is practically instantaneous, and remarkable to observe.

RHYTHMIC MUSIC AND SPEECH

Similar to their problems initiating and maintaining movement, patients with PD, traumatic brain injuries, or stroke may have difficulties articulating words, making their speech slurred and unclear. Sometimes this is due to poor breath support and other times it is a result of challenges with the motor aspects of speech, that is, moving the mouth and tongue to articulate specific sounds. Perception of, as well as the production of, temporal patterns are importantfor both music and speech. Penhune, Zatorre, and Evans (1998), found central control of both motor timing and perceptual timing across modalities to be linked to both the cerebellum and the basal ganglia. The role of the cerebellum in timing is conceptualized not as a clock or counter, but simply as the structure that provides the necessary circuitry for the sensory system to extract
temporal information and for the motor system to learn to produce a precisely timed response. When these structures are not functioning properly, it is nearly impossible to produce clear speech.

Dysarthria is a motor speech problem resulting from dysfunction in the cerebellum and basal ganglia. It occurs in people with stroke, multiple sclerosis, and many other neurological impairments. People with dysarthria have problems in coordinating breath support and articulation. As a result, their speech is unintelligible. For patients with dysarthria, rhythmic cueing of the tempo of the target word or phrase greatly enhances speech intelligibility

(Tomaino & Wilkens, in press). Without cues, speech is slurred. This work supports our ongoing hypothesis that precisely timed stimulation of motor timing pathways through complementary auditory networks allows for enhancement of functioning and greater therapeutic benefit.

In a combined music therapy and speech therapy study (Tomaino & Wilkens, in press) we tested the efficacy of singing and rhythmic self-cueing to enhance speech intelligibility in patients with dysarthria. Each participant was cued to sing familiar song lyrics as they tapped a finger to each syllable they sang. Once this was mastered, we substituted the targeted phrases. At baseline, the average number of intelligible syllables per person was only 3, for example, How are you? After 3 months of working with this group twice a week for 45 minutes, the average number of intelligible syllables increased to 19, a very significant gain for individuals with this kind of difficulty.

Individuals who have had a stroke in Broca's area, an area in the left language region of the brain, have difficultly retrieving words and/or in expressing themselves in words, but despite this, they are able to comprehend speech. This is termed non-fluent aphasia. Interestingly, many people with non-fluent aphasia can sing words to songs with little difficulty. Singing may serve as a priming element for speech, stimulating either peripheral language areas or compensatory areas in the right temporal lobe. For example, some of our non-fluent aphasia patients who have a hard time naming objects can name objects with greater success immediately after they have sung the lyrics to a familiar song.

Research is ongoing to determine the neurological connections between singing and speech in efforts to improve outcomes for persons with this condition (Kim & Tomaino, 2008, p. 8). In the past, this was viewed as a split-brain ability. The thought was that singing is processed in the right temporal lobe; recent research indicates that there is actually bilateral processing of both language and singing (Berlin et al., 1996; Patel, 2005; Patel et al., 2006).

Facial and other rhythmic cues may also have a critical role in the treatment of persons with non-fluent aphasia. To study this, we have been analyzing video from therapy sessions. Besides following the rhythmic cueing of the therapist, during these meetings we've observed that patients are locked on the facial expressions of the therapist, taking in non-verbal cues of oral motor timing and coordination. Research has shown that children learn language through mirroring the facial expressions, tones, and inflections of speech before they are able to use words (Studdert-Kennedy, 1983; Kuhl & Meltzoff, 1996; Lewkowicz, 2003). It was clear to us, as we analyzed these videos, that people with language deficits also rely on other cues to process speech. Building on this observation, in our music therapy sessions various protocols are used, in addition to facial cues, to enhance speech production. These include use of familiar lyrics, speech phrases enhanced by strong melodic contour, novel phrases put to familiar melodies, and speech phrases enhanced by rhythmic cueing. In these cases, the musical cues are eventually removed as independent word retrieval and use of phrases improves.

Singing also can act as a priming element for people who have suffered a stroke. One of my first patients was an elderly man who, after a stroke, stopped speaking. When I met him, he had not spoken for 5 years. He was admitted to a nursing home and became physically rigid and mute. When I began working with him, he would gaze absently into the room, not fixing his sight onto anyone or anything. During my regular sessions on the unit, I played a particular old folk song. I noticed that this man would turn his head towards me only during this song. One time this happened, he and I made eye contact and I sensed that he had a connection to this song—recognized the song and had some sort of personal connection to it. I started to play this song for him everyday, and soon he started to make sounds with his throat, as if he was trying to sing. These sounds soon became the melody of the song. Within a few weeks, with this repetition, he started to sing the actual lyrics, the first words he had spoken in 5 years. When I told his wife that he had started to speak and how this came about, she told me that song we'd been singing was the lullaby he sang to their children every night. His personal connection to the material, with the help of the musical cueing, was enough to help him recover functioning. First came the singing of the words and then the full recovery of speech. It was as if his speech had been locked away for years—he just needed the right stimulation to bring it back.

RHYTHMIC MUSIC AND ATTENTION: TREATMENT OF DEMENTIA

Critically, in persons with dementia, even at late stages, entraining to auditory rhythms is still possible. Such stimulation and engagement impacts attention levels, physical endurance, and interpersonal interactions at the most basic levels. The therapeutic benefits of rhythmic programs to benefit those with dementia have been well documented by Clair (1996) and others. Length of engagement is crucial, as the more time a person with dementia is engaged in an activity, the greater the chance for meaningful response. Repetition is also important. Rhythmic cueing can take advantage of both these elements. Even when patients start a session playing rhythmic patterns that do not directly relate to the rhythmic stimulus provided by the music therapist, they soon entrain to the beat they are hearing. Once this is accomplished, they will continue to tap their synchronous rhythms, with intermittent cueing from the therapist, for as long as the rhythmic stimulus is provided. Change of dynamics and rhythmic patterns throughout the sessions provides enough novelty to increase length of engagement and improve attention over time. With improvement in attention and physical endurance, the carry-over to other aspects of functioning that enhance quality of life become apparent.[4]

RHYTHMIC MUSIC AND RELAXATION

For patients with PD or Huntington's Chorea, excessive involuntary movement or dyskinesia can be slowed by auditory entrainment. In such cases,
the urge to move may impede the need to relax and often disrupts sleep patterns. In these instances, the presentation of slow rhythmic auditory stimuli
can reduce overactive respiration and heart rate and provide the necessary
entrainment for improved relaxation and sleep.

We used this treatment with a patient at our clinic with early onset PD. He
had insomnia with accompanying restless movements that kept him up most
nights. Together, we created a music track that began at a fast tempo and
progressively modulated to slower tempos as the tape went on. The recording
began at a quick tempo to match his feelings of restlessness, and moved into
slower tempos to encourage relaxation and sleep[5]. The duration of the track
was only 20 minutes, but through this method, we were consistently able to
bring him to a low enough state of arousal to let him fall asleep on his own.

FUTURE RESEARCH

Within the field of music therapy, which has been an established profession
in the U.S. since 1950, there is a recognized need for development of more
evidenced-based treatment protocols. The establishment of centers devoted
specifically to studying music therapy applications for people with neurological problems, such as the Institute for Music and Neurologic Function
(IMNF) in New York and The Center for Biomedical Research in Music
(CBRM) in Colorado, has enabled music therapists to receive specialized
training in new methodologies specific to this population.

Both within the field of music therapy and outside it, in particular when
music, that is, rhythm, is being used to effect functioning in a targeted
way, there is a need to standardize protocols as well as identify qualified professionals to provide such treatments. Continued research in both
music therapy and neuroscience is needed to bring new understanding to
and appreciation of the potential impact of auditory entrainment on cognitive and physical functioning. With increased knowledge of how rhythmic
entrainment recruits and stimulatesauditory, motor, and other neural pathways, better therapies can be created to enhance recovery of functioning
after brain trauma and improve maintenance of functioning in those with
progressive diseases.

ACKNOWLEDGMENT

I gratefully acknowledge Gabe Turow for his editorial help and suggestions
to aid in the completion of this paper.

NOTES

1. Certain types of recorded music can be used to induce auditory entrainment, and aid in relaxation and pain reduction. Recordings can be used for reminiscence, speech remediation, and motor cueing. Even when recordings are used, the music therapist makes an assessment of which type of music or component of music will be the most beneficial for the intended goals. Most often these recordings are made after working actively with the client to establish the most appropriate music to use.
2. Research in this area describes the auditory driving of various neural circuits, a process that one would assume is automatic, given the subconscious nature of rhythmic entrainment. As Andrew Neher (1961) suggested, rhythmic music can serve as an entrainment device, possibly driving cortical rhythms as a result of the rhythmic auditory stimulation. Neher defined auditory driving as a general activation of the temporal region, produced by pulsed sound in or near the theta range and suggested that rhythmic entrainment could change brain activity.
3. On a related note, for those who have impaired fine and/or gross motor skills, digital music instruments can be used to reinforce a range of motor function. Electronic keyboards can be adjusted for touch sensitivity allowing for the slightest press on the keys to make a tone. Other devices can be on/off triggers for MIDI-based instruments. One such device is the Soundbeam, an infrared beam that is projected into a space. When the beam is broken, it acts as an On/Off switch to trigger the musical events that were programmed in the Soundbeam controller device. Those events can be chord changes, single tones, or a continuum of sound. As the person moves in space with their arms and hands, he/she hears an auditory signal that reinforces the target movement. This auditory feedback becomes a very strong and powerful therapeutic tool for enabling the reintegration of the perception of and the actual physical range of movement.
4. Music therapy can greatly enhance self-expression in people with neurological impairments. If you can imagine an individual who has lost the ability to move, who has lost the ability to speak, they have in most ways been cut off from other individuals. There is no way for them to relate interpersonally with somebody anymore. And yet we know that meaning can be conveyed in musical expression. We can facilitate music making through digital technologies or active musical improvisations on traditional instruments. In the context of making music together, they have a means of conveying ideas and a way to relate to each other, as part of a community, even if words cannot be spoken. For some of our patients who cannot recover lost functioning, we have a way to allow for expression and meaning. It is incredibly therapeutic and life-affirming.
5. Music therapists refer to matching the tempo or nature of the music with the internal state of the patient as the iso principle. As the patients' mood or arousal changes, changing the stimulation is always crucial.

REFERENCES

Berlin, P., et al. (1996). Recovery from nonfluent aphasia after melodic intonation therapy: A PET study. *Neurology, 47*(6), 1504–1511.

Clair, A. (1996). *Therapeutic uses of music with older adults.* Baltimore, MD: Health Professions Press.

Cohen, N. (1988). The use of superimposed rhythm to decrease the rate of speech in a brain damaged adolescent. *Journal of Music Therapy, 25*, 85–93.

Cohen, N. (1992). The effect of singing instruction on the speech production on neurologically impaired persons. *Journal of Music Therapy, 29*, 87–102.

Condon, W. S. (1975). Multiple response to sound in dysfunctional children. *Journal of Autism and Childhood Schizophrenia, 5*(1), 43.

Gao, W., & Pallas, S. L. (1999). Cross-modal reorganization of horizontal connectivity in auditory cortex without altering thalamocortical projections. *Journal of Neuroscience,15, 19*(18), 7940–7950. PMID: 10479695; UI: 99410775.

Haas, F., Distenfeld, S., & Axen, K. (1986) Effects of perceived musical rhythm on respiratory pattern. *Journal of Applied Physiology, 61*(3), 1185–1191.

Howe, T. E., Lovgreen, B., Cody, F. W., Ashton, V. J., & Oldham, J. A. (2003). Auditory cues can modify the gait of persons with early-stage Parkinson's disease: A method for enhancing Parkinsonian walking performance? *Clinical Rehabilitation, 17*(4), 363–367.

Hurt, C. P., Rice, R. R., McIntosh, G. C., & Thaut, M. H. (1998). Rhythmic auditory stimulation in gait training for patients with traumatic brain injury. *Journal of Music Therapy, 35*(4), 228–241.

Isaichev, S. A., Derevyankin, V. T., Koptelov, YuM., & Sokolov, E. N. (2001). Rhythmic alpha-activity generators in the human EEG. *Neuroscience and Behavioral Physiology, 31*(1), 49–53.

Kim, M., & Tomaino, C. M. (2005). In focus: Cognitive function in people with dementia [German]. In S. Jochims (Ed.), *Music therapy in neurorehabilitation. International concept: Theory and practice.* Germany: Bad Honnef.

Kim, M., & Tomaino, C. M. (2008). Protocol evaluation for effective music therapy for persons with nonfluent aphasia. *Topics in Stroke Rehabilitation.* Nov-Dec, 15(6):555–69.

Kudo, K., Miyazaki, M., Kimura, T., Yamanaka, K., Kadota, H., Hirashima, M., . . . Ohtsuki, T. (2004). Activation and deactivation of the human brain structures between speeded and precisely timed tapping responses to identical stimulus: An fMRI study. *Neuroimage, 22*(3), 1291–1301.

Kuhl, P. K., & Meltzoff, A. N. (1996). Infant vocalizations in response to speech: Vocal imitation and developmental change. *Journal of the Acoustic Society of America, 100*(4, Part1), 2425–2438.

Large, E. W., Fink, P., & Kelso, J. A. S. (2002). Tracking simple and complex sequences. *Psychological Research, 66,* 3–17.

Lewkowicz, D. J. (2003). Learning and discrimination of audiovisual events in human infants: The hierarchical relation between intersensory temporal synchrony and rhythmic pattern cues. *Developmental Psychology, 39*(5), 795–804.

Liberzon, T., & Brown, S. H. (1998). Effects of rhythmic auditory cueing on timing variability of sequential arm movements in Parkinson's disease. *Proceedings Society for Neuroscience, 653,* 18.

McIntosh, G. C., Brown, S. H., Rice, R. R., & Thaut, M. H. (1997). Rhythmic auditory-motor facilitation of gait patterns in patients with Parkinson's disease. *Journal of Neurology, Neurosurgery, and Psychiatry, 62,* 22–26.

Namerow, N. S., Sclabassi, R. J., & Enns, N. F. (1974). Somatosensory responses to stimulus trains: Normative data. *Electroencephalography and Neurophysiology, 37,* 11–21.

Neher, A. (1961). Auditory driving observed with scalp electrodes in normal subjects. *Electroencephalography and Neurophysiology, 13,* 449–451.

Patel, A. D. (2005). The relationship of music to the melody of speech and to syntactic processing disorders in aphasia. *Annals of the New York Academy of Sciences, 1060,* 59–70.

Patel, A. D., & Balaban, E. (2001). Human pitch perception is reflected in the timing of stimulus-related cortical activity. *Nature Neuroscience, 4*(8), 839–844.

Patel, A. D., Iversen, J. R., & Rosenberg, J. C. (2006). Comparing the rhythm and melody of speech and music: The case of British English and French. *Journal of the Acoustical Society of America, 119,* 3034–3047.

Patel, A. D., Peretz, I., Tramo, M., & Raymonde, L. (1998). Processing prosodic and musical patterns: A neuropsychological investigation. *Brain and Language, 61*, 123–144.

Penhume, V. B., Zatorre, R. J., & Evans, A. C. (1998). Cerebellar contributions to motor timing: a PET study of auditory and visual rhythm reproduction. *Journal of Neuroscience, 29(6)*, 752–765.

Repp, B. (2001). Effects of music perception and imagery on sensorimotor synchronization with complex timing patterns. *Annals of the New York Academy of Sciences, 930*, 409–411.

Repp, B. (2002). The embodiment of musical structure: Effects of musical contexts and sensorimotor synchronization with complex timing patterns. In W. Prinz & B. Hommel (Eds.), *Common mechanisms in perception and action: Attention and Performance XIX*. New York: Oxford University Press.

Scheiby, B. B. (2005). Dying alive: A transpersonal analytical music therapy approach for adult clients with chronic progressive neurological diseases. In C. Dileo & J. V. Loewy (Eds.), *Music therapy at the end of life*. Cherry Hill, NJ: Jeffrey Books, pp. 171–187.

Straum, M. (1983). Music and rhythmic stimuli in the rehabilitation of gait disorders and clinical applications. *Journal of Music Therapy, 23*, 56–122.

Studdert-Kennedy, M. (1983). On learning to speak. *Human Neurobiology, 2(3)*, 191–195.

Swartz, K., Walton, J., Crummer, G., Hantz, E., & Frisinia, R. (1992). P3 event-related potentials and performance of healthy older and Alzheimers dementia subjects for musical perception tasks. *Psychomusicology, 11*, 96–118.

Taylor, D. B. (1989). A neurological model for the use of music in the remediation of aphasic disorders. In M. H. Lee (Ed.), *Rehabilitation, music and human wellbeing*. St. Louis, MO: MMB Music.

Thaut, M. H., Kenyon, G. P., Schauer, M. L., & Mclintosh, G. C. (1999). The connection between rhythmicity and brain function. *IEEE Engineering in Medicine and Biology Magazine. 18(2)*, 101–108.

Thaut, M., McIntosh, G., Prassas, S., & Rice, R. (1992). Effect of rhythmic cuing on temporal stride parameters and EMG patterns in normal gait. *Journal of Neurologic Rehabilitation, 6*, 185–190.

Thaut, M. H., McIntoch, G. C., & Rice, R. R. (1997). Rhythmic facilitation of gait training in hemiparetic strokie rehabilitation. *Journal of the Neurological Science, 151(2)*, 207–212.

Thaut, M. H., Miller, R. A., & Schauer, L. M. (1998). Multiple synchronizations strategies in rhythmic sensory motor tasks.: Phase vs. period correction. *Biological Sybernetics, 79*, 241–250.

Tomaino, C. M. (1993). Music and limbic system. In F. Bejjani (Ed.), *Current research in arts and medicine* (pp. 393–398). Chicago: A Capella Books.

Tomaino, C. M. (Ed.). (1998a).Music on their minds: A qualitative study of the effects of using familiar music to stimulate preserved memory function in persons with dementia. Doctoral dissertation, New York University, New York.

Tomaino, C. M. (1998b). (ed). *Clinical Applications of Music in Neurologic Rehabilitation*. MMB, Music: St. Louis.

Tomaino, C., & Wilkens, J. (in press). *Combined music therapy and speech therapy to improve intelligibility in patients with dysarthria*.

Vafaee, M. S., & Gjedde, A. (2004). Spatially dissociated flow-metabolism coupling in brain activation. *Neuroimage, 21(2)*, 507–515.

7 Binaural Beat Stimulation
Altering Vigilance and Mood States

Gabe Turow and James D. Lane

Binaural beat stimulation is a special type of rhythmic auditory stimulation that requires two sine tones, one presented to each ear, differing in frequency by 1 to 30Hz. When played simultaneously, the listener perceives a rhythmic beating sound (amplitude modulation) at a tempo equal to the difference between the frequencies of the two tones. For example, if the left ear hears 100Hz, and the right ear hears 110Hz, the beating will be perceived at 10Hz, or 10 beats per second. Surprisingly, this type of stimulation shows promise as a means to alter brain activity, behavior, and mood. This chapter describes binaural beat stimulation within a research and clinical context and concludes with an account of an experiment conducted by one of the authors (Lane, Kasian, Owens, & Marsh, 1998) to test the effects of binaural beat stimulation on vigilance performance, and mood.

The complexity of music, in terms of its multidimensional and fluid stimulus properties, and the cultural context in which it is experienced, can make it nearly impossible to isolate specific active components that can be investigated for their direct influences on the brain and nervous system. In contrast, binaural beat stimulation provides a method for the rhythmic stimulation of the brain that can be subjected to rigorous scientific scrutiny.

BINAURAL BEATS

The phenomenon of binaural beating is similar in many respects to common acoustic beating that arises from the interference of two sound waves of similar, but slightly different, frequencies. With acoustic beats, when two simple tones of similar frequency are played together, such as those depicted in the top two tracings in Figure 7.1, the sound waveforms interfere with each other to create a complex waveform like that shown in the bottom tracing. The pitch of the complex waveform is the average of the frequencies of the two simple tones. However, the amplitude of the sound that results varies rhythmically, becoming louder and softer, producing a tremolo effect. This happens because as the two simple waveforms interfere

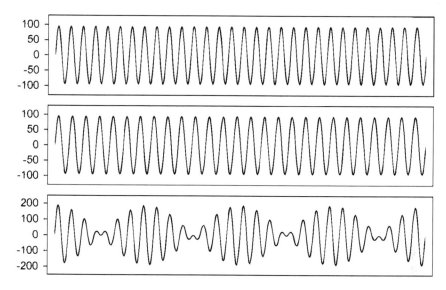

Figure 7.1 Acoustic beating occurs when simple waveforms of similar frequency (top and middle) combine. The resulting complex waveform has a rhythmically modulated amplitude that rises and falls at a frequency equal to the difference between the frequencies of the two simple waveforms.

with each other, they sometimes add together constructively and at other times offset each other.

The tempo of this amplitude modulation, or beating, is always equal to the difference between the frequencies of the original two tones. For example, if the two tones differ in frequency by 15Hz, the amplitude modulation or tremolo will be quite rapid, with a tempo of 15Hz. As the two tones slowly converge to the same pitch, the tremolo slows in frequency until it disappears entirely. When the two simple tones add together maximally, the amplitude of the complex tone is doubled. The amplitude of the complex tone falls to zero when the two simple waveforms combine destructively.

Although binaural beats have a similar sound, they are produced through an entirely different mechanism. Binaural beats occur when two tones of different frequency are presented separately to the left and right ears, as through stereo headphones. Each ear hears only one of the two carrier tones; there is no opportunity for the two waveforms to physically mix in the air, like normal acoustic beats. Despite this separation, the listener perceives a similar kind of tremolo or beat.

The perception of the binaural beat is *created* by the neural processing that occurs when auditory stimuli from the left and right ears are first integrated together (Oster, 1973). This processing takes place in a part of the brainstem called the superior olivary nucleus, which normally functions to integrate contralateral input from the two ears in our perception of sound.

Like the acoustic beat, the binaural beat frequency is equal to the difference between the frequencies of the two carrier tones. Unlike acoustic beats, the amplitude modulation effect or tremolo of binaural beats is fairly subtle. The binaural beat never sounds louder than the carrier tones and the sound of the carrier tones never disappears entirely, as it can for an acoustic beat. The tremolo effect is limited and somewhat muffled.

Binaural beats are best perceived when the carrier tones are about 440Hz (Schwarz & Taylor, 2005). They become less distinct for carriers above that frequency and disappear when frequencies near 3,000Hz. However, carrier tones as low as 90Hz can produce the perceived beat (Oster, 1973). Very slow binaural beats can be perceived, but as the beat frequency increases to about 30Hz, the perception of a distinct beat is replaced by a perceived raspiness in the sound.

Multiple pairs of carrier tones can be combined to produce multiple binaural beats in complex patterns and a background of pink noise, which sounds roughly like rushing water, tends to enhance the perception of the beating. With this type of background noise, it is still possible to perceive the binaural beats even when the carrier tones can barely be heard (Atwater, 2001).

When the same carrier tones are presented to both ears, no binaural beat is created. The causal listener does not notice the difference between the presence and absence of binaural beats, when the sounds are presented within a background of pink noise or other sounds. As a result, it is possible to create credible "placebo" sound recordings that have all the apparent characteristics of the active binaural beat recording, but contain no binaural beats. This is an advantage for research, because it provides a means to isolate experimentally the direct effects of the presence of binaural beats from all other aspects of the subject's experience (Atwater, 2001).

BINAURAL BEAT RESEARCH

In the field of psychoacoustics, binaural beats are a well-documented phenomenon, studied in investigations of sound localization in humans (Oster, 1973) and cats (Kuwada, 1979) and verified encephalographically to induce a very low amplitude frequency following response at various sites in the brains of humans (Smith, Marsh, & Brown, 1975; Smith, Marsh, Greenberg, & Brown, 1978; Yamada, Yamane, & Kodera, 1977; Moushegian, Rupert, & Stillman, 1978; Dobie & Norton, 1980; Schwarz & Taylor, 2005; Wilson & Krishnan, 2005; Karino, 2006) and cats (Wernick & Starr, 1968). In contrast, much less is known about the effects of binaural beat stimulation on free-running EEG in humans.

At issue is whether binaural beat patterns with frequencies comparable to the major frequency bands of the human EEG (beta, alpha, theta, and delta) can increase rhythmic electrical activity of the brain in these frequency bands. Atwater (2001) exposed subjects to a 45-minute program that included alpha and delta frequency binaural beats, with the presence of the alpha stimulus decreasing over time and the presence of the delta stimulus increasing. Corresponding changes were observed in the EEG activity, as alpha frequency activity decreased during the session and delta frequency activity increased. No systematic changes were observed when a placebo program was presented. A small pilot study by another group (Brady & Stevens, 2000) found that a 20-minute program of EEG theta frequency binaural beat stimulation produced increases in EEG theta activity during the session. However, a larger, more controlled replication study (Stevens et al., 2003) found that theta EEG activity increased similarly over time in both the experimental (theta) and placebo groups, a result that casts doubt on the specific effects of the binaural beats, and suggests that earlier effects may have been due simply to the development of drowsiness over time.

Much of what is known about the clinical applications of binaural beats comes from anecdotal reports by its users and published case studies of its effects (Monroe, 1982; Hutchison, 1986; Atwater, 1988; Russell, 2004), but some peer-reviewed studies are available. Binaural beats have been shown to decrease acute preoperative anxiety compared to controls (Padmanabhan, Hildreth, & Laws, 2005), reduce general anxiety (Le Scouarnec et al., 2001; Wahbeh et al., 2007), alter mood (Wahbeh et al., 2007), and reduce the need for anaesthesia during surgery (Kliempt, Ruta, Ogston, Landeck, & Martay, 1999; Lewis, Osborn, & Roth, 2004). Effects on hypnotic susceptibility were reported in the same pilot study mentioned previously, when 3, 20-minute sessions of theta binaural beat stimulation apparently increased susceptibility in medium or low, but not high-hypnotizable subjects (Brady & Stevens, 2000). However, the larger replication study (Stevens et al., 2003) that included only low and medium hypnotizable subjects and provided more exposure to binaural beats (4 hours over 2 weeks), did not find any changes in hypnotic susceptibility.

ROBERT MONROE

Robert Monroe (1915 to 1995) was the first person to extensively investigate the effects of binaural beat stimulation on humans and to develop specific applications for clinical use (Monroe, 1982). In the 1950s, Monroe was a radio producer in New York City. Familiar with sound and recording technology, he and colleagues explored the use of audio signals to alter states of arousal and attention. Following the publication of the Oster article in *Scientific American* (Oster, 1973), his group began to employ binaural beats to elicit changes in subjective experience and consciousness. In 1974, he established The Monroe Institute, a non-profit research and educational center located in rural Virginia. The Monroe Institute is now internationally recognized as a resource for binaural-beat research, residential training, and the development of binaural beat stimulation applications for health and personal growth. Monroe continued working with binaural beats for more than three decades (documented in three books: Monroe, 1971, 1985, 1994) until his death in 1995.

In his many years of research (described in: Stockton, 1990; Russell, 2004, 2007) Monroe seldom used binaural beats by themselves, due to the blandness (and somewhat grating nature) of repeated sine tones. He found that embedding the beats in other sounds, like randomized low-frequency pink noise, ameliorated this effect. Monroe called his audio programs Hemi-Sync, based on an observation that listening to binaural beat patterns often created states of EEG coherence between the left and right hemispheres (an observation that currently lacks proper scientific validation).

The binaural beat patterns used to alter states of arousal and attention are those with frequencies within the range of normal human brainwaves. In the years of developmental work, Monroe and others found that higher frequency binaural beat patterns, within the EEG beta frequency band, tended to produce states of alertness, arousal, and enhanced mental focus. They also kept the listener from falling asleep. In contrast, patterns with lower frequencies in the alpha, theta, or delta bands seemed to reduce arousal and produce states of relaxed attention, drowsiness, or sleep. Given the known relationship between EEG activity and states of arousal and attention (Rechtschaffen & Kales, 1968), these experimental observations led his group to the hypothesis that rhythmic binaural beat stimulation might, under appropriate conditions, shift or entrain EEG activity toward the frequency of the binaural beat. This hypothesis echoes the logic of the auditory driving hypothesis, described in Chapters 1–3 of this book.[1]

MECHANISMS OF ACTION

There has been speculation about the specific brain mechanisms that might be involved in the transfer of binaural beat stimulation to altered EEG activity. Monroe and colleagues initially suggested that the repetitive stimulation provided by the binaural beat produced a constant signal from the auditory integration centers that was conducted throughout the brain volume to influence EEG activity (Atwater, 2001). It is possible to measure a low amplitude electrical signal on the scalp that mirrors the waveform of the binaural beat (discussed previously in Binaural Beat Research). This signal is called a frequency following response, and it does indicate the volume conduction of the binaural beat signal throughout the brain. *However, this initial explanation was later rejected, because the frequency following response involved electrical signals that were very small in amplitude and thus unlikely to dominate EEG activity.*

The current hypothesis suggests that the binaural beat signal influences brain activity through the brain's reticular activating system, a network of brain regions that control central nervous system arousal (Atwater, 2001).

Under suitable conditions, especially in the absence of other more dramatic influences, the constant stimulus of the binaural beat is hypothesized to exert an effect on the reticular activating system, which in turn, stimulates the thalamus and cortex to alter arousal states and states of consciousness, perhaps through the release of neurotransmitters.

This hypothesis is speculation at this point, but remains plausible. The reticular activating system is known to integrate sensory inputs from various sources and to exert powerful control over brain activity related to states of consciousness, especially those related to arousal. This seems to be the most likely mechanism by which a relatively low level auditory signal (compared to an intense stimulus like loud drumming) could produce widespread effects on consciousness.

APPLICATIONS

Existing clinical applications of binaural beats fall into two categories, a dichotomy that may be useful in the development and testing of new applications. Many applications take advantage of the presumed effects of binaural beats to increase or decrease the level of arousal within the brain and nervous system. Binaural beat programs of this type have been employed to maintain alertness, to treat attention deficit disorder (ADD), to relax, to fall asleep, to meditate, or to manage pain (Lane et al., 1998; Kliempt et al., 1999; Le Scouarnec et al., 2001; Russell, 2004; Padmanabhan et al., 2005; Wahbeh et al., 2007). People listen to these programs whenever the desired effect is sought. In contrast, the second category of application uses binaural beats to produce a special state of heightened suggestibility, somewhat like a hypnotic state (Brady & Stevens, 2000; Stevens et al., 2003). This state is used with verbal suggestions to teach specific mind/body skills. Once the skills are learned, the binaural beat program is no longer needed to produce the desired effects (Russell, 2004).

Binaural beat patterns are seldom used alone in these applications. They are usually combined with music or other sounds and with verbal instructions or guidance that are thought to enhance the outcome. The resulting recorded audio program is then distributed for use on tape cassettes or CDs. *The authors of this chapter cannot confirm that binaural beats are effective when used for these purposes*, but the results of the following study suggest several interesting possibilities.

BINAURAL AUDITORY BEATS AFFECT
VIGILANCE, PERFORMANCE, AND MOOD

At the urging of a Duke pre-med student Stefan Kasian working in my lab, I (JDL) began a project to explore the behavioral and mood effects of binaural beat stimulation with a team of researchers that included faculty colleagues Gail Marsh from the Department of Psychiatry and Behavioral Sciences, Duke University Medical Center, and Justine Owens from the Center for the Study of Complementary and Alternative Therapies at the School of Nursing, University of Virginia at Charlottesville, Virginia. We set out to test the claim that playing higher frequency (16 to 24Hz) binaural beats could improve attention and performance in the classroom (Russell, 2004). Specifically, we wanted to test whether binaural beats by themselves could influence attention and cognitive performance under rigorous experimental conditions (Lane et al., 1998).

We discussed the project with the staff of The Monroe Institute, who had the most practical experience working with binaural beats. They reminded us that binaural beat stimulation was only one component of the audio programs they typically used. In their experience, the other sounds, music, verbal guidance, and instruction all contributed to the effects that were observed, and the expectations and cooperation of the listener were critical to the outcome that was achieved with the program. They emphasized that binaural beats by themselves might have only a limited effect on consciousness. Despite these concerns, we decided that the critical issue was to establish the validity of the unique component in these programs, to demonstrate that binaural beats by themselves could affect brain activity, arousal, and attention, without any of the other components and, perhaps, even without the listener's expectation of what should happen. *The idea that listening to simple tones on headphones could alter brain functioning seemed almost impossible and was certainly an unlikely hypothesis for our group and most of our colleagues at the time.*

We understood that only the most rigorous, well-controlled experiment would be able to produce the kind of evidence that was needed to persuade a skeptical scientific audience. So we designed a study that we hoped might provide convincing evidence of binaural beat effects. Because we knew that a single binaural beat pattern might have only modest effects, we decided to contrast two binaural beat patterns that we expected to have opposite effects (slow beats in the theta/delta EEG range versus fast beats in the beta EEG range). Potentially, this would create a difference between conditions that would be easier to detect than if we were looking for a difference between a single pattern and a "placebo" control.

A major concern was that reviewers of our work would assume that the reported influences of binaural beats were simply placebo effects, produced not by the sound patterns themselves but by the listeners' expectations and by other components of the experimental protocol. Subjects might become sleepy or alert because they expected to, or because the musical or instructional content of a program suggested it. We therefore chose to use binaural beat patterns without music or instruction. In addition, we kept the presence of the binaural beat patterns secret from the subjects. Because they were "blind" to the experimental manipulation, there could be no expectation about what should happen. Although deception of human subjects is seldom acceptable, this specific deception was approved by our Institutional Review Board for the protection of human subjects as a necessary feature of the study. Together these choices created the basis for a study could provide the strongest possible evidence that binaural beat stimulation could (or doesn't) have direct effects on brain activity or consciousness. If we did indeed observe the predicted effects, we knew that such a test might well underestimate the real effects of binaural beats as they were normally used (given the lack of expectation effects, etc.), but such a test would be a critical step in gaining scientific acceptance of the fact that such simple recorded sounds could have distinct, and meaningful, effects.

METHODS

The study included three different recorded audio programs. For our experimental test, we incorporated two contrasting binaural beat patterns, one that had previously been associated with alertness and arousal versus another associated with drowsiness and the onset of sleep. Each of these patterns contained multiple carrier tones that produced two binaural beat frequencies in either the EEG beta band (16 and 24Hz) or the EEG theta/ delta band (1.5 and 4Hz). The third program contained the same carrier tones, but included no binaural beats. All three programs contained the same pink noise background that made the carrier tones barely perceptible. As a result, all three programs sounded identical to the subjects

Each participant took part in three different tests, listening to each of the three recorded programs. The first test session was used to acquaint each subject with experimental procedures while listening to the program without binaural beats (only pink noise and carrier tones). The experimental test conditions were presented next, with the order of presentation for the beta and theta/delta binaural beat programs randomly varied among the study participants to prevent any systematic bias that could result from the order in which the patterns were presented. It bears repeating that study participants were kept blind throughout the study to the true purpose of the experiment. They were told that the sounds they heard during testing were intended only to block out ambient noises. They were unaware of the presence of binaural beats. In addition, the experimenter who conducted each test session was unaware of which pattern was being presented, to eliminate this source of possible influence on participants.

VIGILANCE TASK

We attempted to find an experimental task that would potentially reveal the expected changes in alertness versus drowsiness. We decided that a sustained vigilance task, where attention has to be maintained continuously under very monotonous conditions, would provide a good opportunity to see the effects of binaural beats on arousal. Other studies have shown that sustained attention and vigilance performance are affected by changes in the level of arousal in the brain and that these changes can enhance or impair the ability to keep attention focused on this kind of task (Beatty, Greenberg, Deibler, & O'Hanlon, 1974).

For our test of vigilance and sustained attention, study participants monitored a computer display continuously for 30 minutes. Capital letters were displayed sequentially, one at a time, for 1/10 of a second, at a rate of 1 per second, or 60 letters per minute. Whenever the observer saw the same letter repeated in the series, he or she pressed a computer key to respond to this target. These targets were rare, only happening 6 times each minute, and the task continued uninterrupted for 30 minutes. Because the letters were presented only briefly, subjects had to pay constant attention. They also had to keep track of each letter as it appeared to compare it to the next. Task performance was judged by the number of targets detected, and the number of incorrect responses made when no target was presented ("false alarms").

To make the task more difficult, subjects worked in a quiet, darkened room. They wore headphones that blocked out ambient noise and presented the binaural tones within a background of pink noise. Under such conditions, this task gets monotonous very quickly; it becomes more difficult to stay focused over time. If a subject became drowsy, he would be likely to miss a target, or get confused and respond when no target was presented.

Before and after the vigilance task, participants completed a questionnaire called the Profile of Mood States (POMS; McNair, Lorr, & Droppleman, 1992), in order to assess changes in moods including anger, confusion, depression, fatigue, tension/anxiety, and vigor. We used this questionnaire because we wanted to know how the vigilance task made the subjects feel, and whether the binaural beats altered their experience in any way. A group of 29 healthy participants, mostly college students, completed the study.

RESULTS

Measures of performance on the sustained attention vigilance task showed that there were clear differences between the high and low frequency binaural beat conditions, consistent with our predictions. Figure 7.2 shows the average number of targets that were detected in each condition and the average number of false alarm responses. More targets were detected in the high frequency or beta stimulation condition (gray bar), with fewer false alarms, than in the low frequency or theta/delta stimulation condition (black bar).

When study participants listened to the beta EEG frequency binaural beat patterns, they detected an average of 153.5 of the 180 targets. When they listened to theta/delta stimulation, they only detected 147.6 targets, a

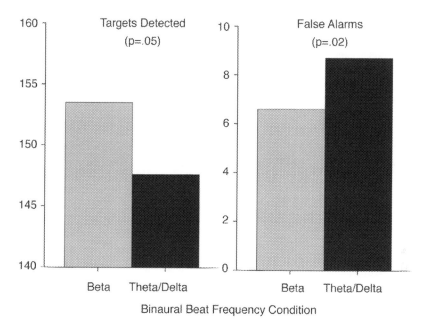

Figure 7.2 Target detection graphs. Results showed clear differences between the two binaural beat patterns. Vigilance performance was measured using a 30-minute test with 180 targets.

small difference that was statistically significant. False alarms, which could represent confusion and inattention during the task, were fewer when participants listened to the beta pattern, with an average of 6.6 false alarms compared to 8.7 when listening to the theta/delta pattern. This modest difference was also statistically significant. Performance on the vigilance task was better on both measures when subjects heard the beta-frequency binaural beat patterns, even though the subjects were completely unaware

Table 7.1 Mood Changes During Testing

Changes in mood from before to after the 30 minute Vigilance Task

	Beta	Theta/Delta	Difference	*p-value*
Change in Confusion/ Bewilderment	0.9	1.9	-1.0	*p*=.01
Change in Fatigue/ Inertia	2.3	3.6	-1.3	*p*=.05

of the presence of the beats during testing. This was consistent with our hypothesis that the beta frequencies would enhance alertness and sustained attention, compared to the slower frequency stimuli.

The two patterns also had effects on mood consistent with our expectations. As Table 7.1 shows, performing the 30-minute vigilance task produced increases in scores on the POMS scales for "confusion/bewilderment", which reflects mental fatigue or fuzziness, and "fatigue/inertia". The task made subjects feel both mentally and physically tired. However, these increases were significantly smaller when subjects listened to the beta frequency binaural beat pattern than when they listened to the theta/delta pattern. The pattern that we thought would enhance alertness, and which did enhance performance, was associated with less mental and physical fatigue at the end of the task.

CONCLUSIONS

This study demonstrated that different patterns of binaural beat stimulation by themselves produced alterations in both cognitive performance and mood. These results demonstrate that binaural beat patterns can alter brain function, even if the listener is unaware of their presence. One might argue that these differences, though statistically significant, were in fact quite small; the authors would not disagree. *However, the importance of these results is not the size of the difference, but the fact that we could detect any difference that can only be attributed to the presence of the different patterns of binaural beats.* Experimental controls prevented any extraneous influence, including the expectations of the participant or experimenter. We probably could create larger effects by combining the binaural beats with other sounds or with instructions that encourage the participation of the listener in the experience. That is how these stimuli are normally used—but we showed that such manipulations are not necessary to alter cognitive performance and perceived mood.

The design of this study does not give us the opportunity to compare each of the treatments with a "no-treatment" condition. We cannot say whether either pattern had effects different from no pattern at all. That is an important question, but it was not the objective of this study. Neither did this study include measures of brain activity like EEG, which were not available to us at the time. These measures are certainly important for the continued study of binaural beats. But again, they were not critical to our attempt to show that these simple audio signals could alter cognitive performance and mood in a manner consistent with hypothesized shifts in arousal levels within the brain and nervous system.

This study was a first step towards establishing the scientific validity of binaural beat auditory stimulation for the manipulation of brain function and consciousness. Although it was a small step, publication of these results in a peer-reviewed scientific journal provided a foundation for future research to advance our understanding of the application of binaural beats.

FUTURE RESEARCH

We can offer several recommendations for future basic science studies of binaural beat stimulation. There is a critical need for controlled experimental studies to confirm the basic assumptions that binaural beat stimulation can affect brain function and consciousness. The torrent of anecdotal evidence cannot by itself overcome the skepticism that simple audio signals can alter brain function, attention, arousal, and mood. This basic scientific research is important in its own right, but it is also critical for the development of clinical and self-improvement applications. We have tried to interest colleagues at Duke University Medical Center in tests of clinical applications of binaural beats, but they find it implausible that simply listening to a tape or CD could have clinical benefit. They want first to see hard evidence that these stimuli can affect consciousness. Only basic science studies can provide this.

The research that should come next will test whether binaural beat stimulation can affect brain functioning and define the different ways that it can do so. EEG studies of the brain's electrical activity will be useful, especially to test the hypothesis that these auditory signals entrain specific EEG frequencies. However, studies of cognitive performance, such as the one outlined here, will also provide useful evidence to support practical applications. For example, our evidence of enhanced attention during vigilance suggests that these binaural beats could be potentially useful in the treatment of ADD. Pilot clinical trials would also be useful at this time, perhaps aimed at the applications where anecdotal evidence is the strongest.

In closing, binaural beats have two strengths that recommend them as a method for altering brain and nervous system functioning. For research, it is critically important that binaural beat studies can include a true placebo control, like the "sugar pill" used in drug studies, and that it is possible to keep subjects blind to the treatment they are receiving. This is the only way that the true and specific effects of a treatment can be determined. To properly investigate the use of binaural beats for clinical work, the context and circumstances that will support and encourage these influences must be examined and bolstered by neuroscientific study of dynamic brain activity and cognitive performance. Investigations of the behavioral and emotional responses that demonstrate the expression of underlying neural processes will also be crucial. The second strength relates to potential clinical applications. The fact that binaural beats are audio stimuli, which can be presented on tape cassette, CD, or MP3, is very useful. Not only do they represent a cost-effective therapeutic modality, but they can potentially be used during many different activities, played through headphones. This kind of flexibility is not available with all forms of rhythmic stimulation.

NOTES

1. For example, stereophonic presentation of 200Hz and 209Hz tones to the left and right ears respectively, creates the perception of a 9Hz binaural beat. Hypothetically, if this stimulus were maintained for several minutes, the EEG would be entrained to produce an increase in activity at 9Hz. The increase in EEG activity at 9Hz, within the alpha band (8–12Hz), would then elicit the subjective state of awake relaxation typically associated with increased alpha activity (Lindsley, 1952; Brown, 1977). The few free-running EEG studies on binaural beats have observed a general correspondence between binaural beat frequency and brainwave states, such as increases or decreases in alpha or theta band activity (Brady & Stevens, 2000; Atwater, 2001), but the specific correspondence between binaural beat and EEG frequency predicted by this theory needs further empirical documentation to establish it.

REFERENCES

Atwater, F. H. (1988). *The Monroe Institute's Hemi-Sync process: A theoretical perspective*. Faber, VA: Monroe Institute. Reprinted at: http://www.monroeinstitute.org/journal/binaural-beats-and-the-regulation-of-arousal-levels

Atwater, F. (2001). *Binaural beats and the regulation of arousal levels*. Proceedings of the IANS 11th Forum on New Arts and Science by the International Association on New Science, 1612 Windsor Court, Fort Collins, CO 80526.

Beatty, J., Greenberg, A., Deibler, W. P., & O'Hanlon, J. F. (1974). Operant control of occipital theta rhythm affects performance in a radar monitoring task. *Science, 183*(127), 871–873.

Brady, B., & Stevens, L. (2000). Binaural-beat induced theta EEG activity and hypnotic susceptibility. *American Journal of Clinical Hypnosis, 43*(1), 53–69.

Brown, B. B. (1977). *Stress and the art of Biofeedback*. New York: Bantam Books.

Dobie, R. A., & Norton, S. J. (1980). Binaural interaction in human auditory evoked potentials. *Electroencephalography and Clinical Neurophysiology, 49*, 303–313.

Hutchison, M. (1986). *Megabrain: New tools and techniques for brain growth and mind expansion*. New York: Beech Tree Books.

Karino, S., Yumoto, M., Itoh, K., Uno, A., Yamakawa, K., Sekimoto, S., & Kaga, K. (2006). Neuromagnetic responses to binaural beat in human cerebral cortex. *Journal of Neurophysiology, 96*(4), 1927–1938.

Kliempt, P., Ruta, D., Ogston, S., Landeck, A., & Martay, K. (1999). Hemispheric synchronization during anaesthesia: A double blind randomized trial using audiotapes for intra-operative nociception control. *Anaesthesia, 54*(8), 769–773.

Kuwada, S., Yin, C., & Wickesberg, R. E. (1979). Response of cat inferior colliculus neurons to binaural beat stimuli: Possible mechanisms for sound localization. *Science, 206*(4418), 586–588.

Lane, J. D., Kasian, S. J., Owens, J. E., & Marsh, G. R. (1998). Binaural auditory beats affect vigilance performance and mood. *Physiology and Behavior, 63*(2), 249–252.

Le Scouarnec, R. P., Poirier, R. M., Owens, J. E., Gauthier, J., Taylor, A. G., & Foresman, P. A. (2001). Use of binaural beat tapes for treatment of anxiety: A pilot study of tape preference and outcomes. *Alternative Therapy Health Medicine, 7*(1), 58–63.

Lewis, A. K., Osborn, I. P., & Roth, R. (2004). The effect of hemispheric synchronization on intraoperative analgesia. *Anesthesia & Analgesia, 98*, 533–536.

Lindsley, D. (1952). Psychological phenomena and the electroencephalogram. *Electroencephalogr Clininical Neurophysiology Supplement, 4*(4), 443–456.

McNair, D. M., Lorr, M., & Droppleman, L. F. (1992). *EdITS manual for the profile of mood states.* San Diego: EdITS.

Monroe, R. (1971). *Journeys out of the body.* Garden City, NY: Doubleday.

Monroe, R. (1982). *The hemi-sync process.* Monroe Institute Bulletin, PR31380H. Nellysford, VA.

Monroe, R. (1985). *Far journeys.* New York: Doubleday.

Monroe, R. (1994). *Ultimate journey.* New York: Doubleday.

Moushegian, G., Rupert, A. L., & Stillman, R. D. (1978). Evaluation of frequency-following potentials in man: Masking and clinical studies. *Electroencephalography and Clinical Neurophysiology, 45*, 711–718.

Oster, G. (1973). Auditory beats in the brain. *Scientific American, 229*, 94–102.

Padmanabhan, R., Hildreth, A. J., & Laws, D. (2005). A prospective, randomised, controlled study examining binaural beat audio and pre-operative anxiety in patients undergoing general anaesthesia for day case surgery. *Anaesthesia, 60*(9), 874–877.

Rechtschaffen, A., & Kales, A. (Eds.). (1968). *A manual of standardized terminology, techniques and scoring system for sleep stages of human subjects.* UCLA, Los Angeles: BIS/BRI.

Russell, R. (2004). *Focusing the whole brain: Transforming your life with hemispheric synchronization.* Charlottesville, VA: Hampton Roads Publishing Company, Inc.

Russell, R. (2007). *The journey of Robert Monroe: From out of body explorer to consciousness pioneer.* Charlottesville, VA: Hampton Roads Publishing Company, Inc.

Schwarz, D. W., & Taylor, P. (2005). Human auditory steady state responses to binaural and monaural beats. *Clinical Neurophysiology, 116*(3), 658–668.

Smith, J. C., Marsh, J. T., & Brown, W. S. (1975). Far-field recorded FFR's: Evidence for the locus of brainstem sources. *Electroencephalography and Clinical Neurophysiology, 39*, 465–472.

Smith, J. C., Marsh, J. T., Greenberg, S., & Brown, W. S. (1978). Human auditory frequency-following responses to a missing fundamental. *Science, 201*, 639–641.

Stevens, L., Haga, Z., Queen, B., Brady, B., Adams, D., Gilbert, J., . . . McManus, P. (2003). Binaural beat induced theta EEG activity and hypnotic susceptibility: Contradictory results and technical considerations. *American Journal of Clinical Hypnosis, 45*(4), 295–309.

Stockton, B. (1990). *Catapult: The biography of Robert A. Monroe.* Norfolk, VA: Donning Co.

Wahbeh, H., Calabrese, C., & Zwickey, H. (2007). Binaural beat technology in humans: A pilot study to assess psychologic and physiologic effects. *Journal of Alternative and Complementary Medicine, 13*(1), 25–32.

Wahbeh, H., Calabrese, C., Zwickey, H., & Zajdel, D. (2007). Binaural beat technology in humans: A pilot study to assess neuropsychologic, physiologic, and electroencephalographic effects. *Journal of Alternative and Complementary Medicine, 13*(2), 199–206.

Wernick, J. S., & Starr, A. (1968). Binaural interaction in the superior olivary complex of the cat: An analysis of field potentials evoked by binaural-beat stimuli. *Journal of Neurophysiology, 31*(3), 428–441.

Wilson, J. R., & Krishnan, A. (2005). Human frequency-following responses to binaural masking level difference stimuli. *Journal of American Academic Audiology, 16(3)*, 184–195.

Yamada, O., Yamane, H., & Kodera, K. (1977). Simultaneous recordings of the brain stem response and the frequency-following response to low-frequency tone. *Electroencephalography and Clinical Neurophysiology, 43*, 362–370.

8   Audio-Visual Stimulation
Research and Clinical Practice

Thomas Budzynski, Helen K. Budzynski, Leslie H. Sherlin, and Hsin Yi Tang

INTRODUCTION

Audio-visual stimulation combines flashing light stimulation with rhythmic auditory stimulation synchronized to the same frequency. AVS can be operated from a computer or with a portable cassette-tape-sized device. The user wears headphones and a set of glasses outfitted with small colored light emitting diodes (LEDs). The computer and portable units feature a wide variety of programs and settings to vary stimulation parameters, and these parameters can be controlled by the user or a separate operator.

Our (Budzynski et al.) interest in AVS began in the early 1980s, as AVS units became became commercially available. We slowly began to employ these units in our neurofeedback clinic, using AVS as a form of relaxing stimulation to begin each neurofeedback session. Our interest increased in AVS as clinical research began to emerge, and as we discovered that some of our clients with anxiety were able to eliminate their use of anti-anxiety medication (Librium) with twice weekly sessions of theta frequency (4–7Hz) photic stimulation. Over the next decade, Dr. Budzynski's interest in this modality continued to grow. He published two compendiums of research and clinical applications of AVS in 1991 and has continued his research and clinical work since then[1].

As time went on, evidence for the efficacy of AVS as a therapeutic intervention continued to build. Of particular interest, in 1993, Carter and Russell published a pilot investigation of auditory and visual entrainment of brainwave activity in learning disabled boys (see Chapter 9) and Russell (1997) later published a larger study of an EEG-driven audio-visual stimulation unit used to enhance intellectual functioning in children and adults. In 2003, Dave Siever authored three important articles on AVS in Biofeedback. Siever discussed the history and physiological mechanisms of AVS, dental studies on TMJ, and relaxation with AVS (Solomon, 1985; Anderson, 1989), and the uses of AVS to modify states of attention and learning abilities (Siever, 2003).

COGNITIVE PERFORMANCE ENHANCEMENT
IN COLLEGE STUDENTS

In the early '90s, anecdotal reports from Korea noted that many students were getting an exam edge on other students through the use of small, inexpensive AVS units. Studies on peak alpha frequency (PAF), as well as that of high band alpha (10–12Hz), showed that increased PAF and magnitude in the high band alpha correlated with better performance on various IQ and cognitive performance tests (Giannitrapani, 1969; Giannitrapani, 1988; Anokhin & Vogel,1996; Jausovec, 1996; Klimesch, Doppelmayr, Pachinger, & Ripper, 1997). It seemed reasonable to infer that heightening peak alpha frequencies and increasing the power of high band alpha might be accomplished by means of AVS and/or neurofeedback, and perhaps would improve cognitive performance.

In 1998, we studied a group of 34 subjects (primarily University of Washington grad students) with an average age of 25 to see if light/sound stimulation would result in alpha changes. The findings showed that AVS of 14Hz square waves (Biolight System, from Synetic Systems) tended to increase A3/A1 (High/Low Alpha ratio where A1 = the magnitude of the band 7–9Hz and A3 = the magnitude of the band 11–13Hz, see Figure 8.1).[2] Furthermore, repeated measures showed that A3/A1 continued to increase even at the 20-minutes-post-stimulus point. A similar effect is shown in Figure 8.2 where PAF, as measured at Cz, continued to increase even at P20 minutes. These observations however, were not carried on for more than 20 minutes post stimulation (Budzynski & Tang, 1998).

Most subjects reported that right after the stimulation they felt slightly disoriented, however, after a brief period of roughly 10–15 minutes, they experienced an increase in cognitive clarity over that which they normally felt. More recent studies, primarily carried out by the Klimesch group (Vogt, Klimesch, & Doppelmayr, 1998; Doppelmayr, et al., 2005; Doppelmayr, Klimesch, Hodlmoser, Sauseng, & Gruber, 2005; Klimesch et al., 2005; Sauseng, Klimesch, Schabus, & Doppelmayer, 2005), have buttressed the idea that individuals with more power in the high alpha band (10–12Hz) achieve better academic performance than those with less high alpha band power. We ran a follow-up study in 1999 at the Counseling Center at Western Washington University (WWU) to continue to investigate the effects of AVS on cognition (Budzynski, Jordy, Kogan Budzynski, Tang, & Claypoole, 1999). Students worried about their academic performance who had sought help from the Counseling Center were targeted for this research project. All volunteers had to have completed at least one quarter at WWU so that we had a baseline GPA. Half of these students were randomly assigned to an experimental group (E) whereas the other half constituted a waiting control group (C). All volunteers were told that they could continue being seen at the Counseling Center. Most of the waiting controls continued the counseling sessions but very few of the E group did so. Based on our

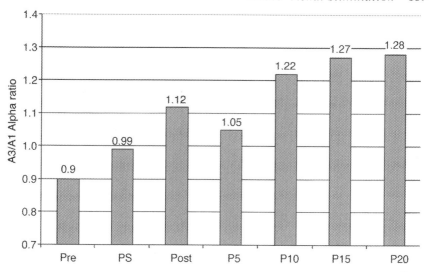

Figure 8.1 Photic simulation and changes in A3/A1 Alpha ratio. PS F = 14Hz, n = 34.

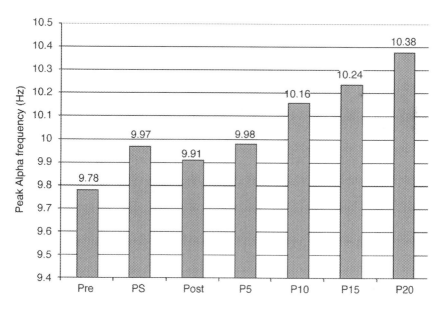

Figure 8.2 Photic stimulation and peak Alpha frequency. PS F = 14Hz, n = 34.

research with varying frequency stimulation, we designed a protocol that would alternate between 22Hz and 14Hz. The AVS device we used for this study (Biolight, Synetic Systems) also had electrodermal response (EDR) feedback capability. It could present a tone that would decrease with EDR level. Participants in the E group were asked to lower the tone as they were presented with 20 minutes of photic stimulation.

A total of 8 participants in each group constituted the final number who completed both pre and post testing. A large number of variables were generated from this study, including measures of EDR, finger temperature, heart rate, and 2 EEG sites, F7 and F8. Pre and post testing included a PSP or Psychophysiological Stress Profile (Relaxation-Stress-Recovery; Budzynski & Stoyva, 1984), stress tests which included subtests of the WAIS and WRAT, aswell as Digit Span and Digit Symbol. Finally, grade point averages (GPAs) were gathered from the academic quarters before training began, during training, and post training. The mean post–pre GPA differences are shown in Figure 8.3. These pre–post GPA differences tell us that the AVS/EDR feedback training did indeed improve academic performance, as the Korean students claimed.

THE AUDIO IN AVS

Certain audio signals, such as binaural tones, seem to have EEG entrainment capability, although this need to be verified with basic research.[3] Commercial AVS units have employed binaural tones, clicks, pulsed sounds, and even music with embedded binaural tones. Binaural tones seem to produce a stronger effect when they are barely above the auditory threshold.

A binaural tone sequence of beta to alpha frequencies (15-10-9-8-10Hz) was incorporated into a self-help cassette/CD ("Revitalizer"[4]) by the first author.

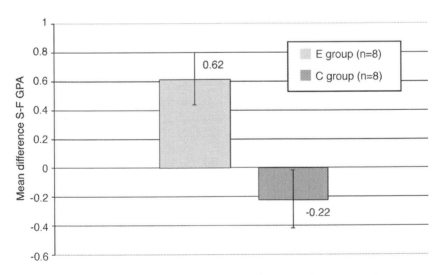

Figure 8.3   Mean GPA post–pre differences, Fall 1997 and Spring 1998.

A quantitative electroencephalogram (QEEG) brainmap generated when a subject was listening to this cassette showed a compressed spectral array (CSA) which portrayed the subject's peak alpha frequency tracking the faint binaural tone. Clearly more research is necessary to understand the effects of the different components of AVS. In general, the addition of sound to the photic stimulation would appear to strengthen the effect of the AVS phenomenon.[5] With the advent of QEEG, fMRI, and SPECT scanning we should be able to test the effects of these stimuli variations much more accurately than in the past.

REGIONAL CEREBRAL BLOOD FLOW AND AVS

Numerous studies have documented the decrease in regional cerebral blood flow (rCBF) in elderly people with ARCD (Melamed, Lavy, Bentin, Cooper, & Rinot, 1980; Gur, Gur, Obrist, Skolnick, & Reivich, 1987; Mints, Litinyenko, & Bachinskaya, 1987–1988; Heiss, Pawlik, Holthoff, Kessler, & Szelies, 1992; Wszolek, Herkes, Lagerlund, & Kokmen, 1992; Meyer, Terayama, & Takashima, 1993; Wyper, 1993; Alexander, Prohovnik, Stern, & Mayeux, 1994; Waldemar, 1995; Celsis et al., 1997; Nagahama et al., 1997). Age Related Cognitive Decline (ARCD), a common condition in aging adults, is characterized by generalized lowered functioning in the domains of short term memory, delayed recall, difficulty in word finding, speed of processing, and sustained attention, among other issues (Peterson, Smith, Kokmen, Ivnid, & Tangalos, 1992). Importantly, when we began examining this literature in the early '90s, we found that AVS appeared to be a good technique to alter patterns of rCBF, and therefore, might be a good treatment for ARCD.

Fox and Raichle's 1985 study demonstrated that CBF in the striate cortex was increased as much as 29% at a frequency of 7.8Hz of photic stimulation. In their publication in 1988 Fox and colleagues described a 50% increase in striate CBF and increased glucose uptake with little change in oxygen consumption during photic stimulation as measured with positron emission tomography (PET). Sappey-Mariner's (1992) research using MRI showed increased cerebral visual cortex blood lactate, indicating non-oxidative glucose consumption by an average of 250%, in the first 6 minutes of 2Hz photic stimulation.

Mentis and colleagues (1997) used an alternating pattern flash at frequencies of 0–14Hz to study effects on the rCBF in various parts of the brain. They found that the left middle temporal area (BA 19/37) was activated at 1Hz and the left anterior cingulate was activated biphasically at 2–14Hz with a maximum at 4Hz, whereas the right frontal, middle and anterior cingulate, and right superior temporal areas decreased monotonically in rCBF with increasing flash frequency from 0–14Hz.

Interestingly, Mentis and colleagues (1997) and also Rapoport and Grady (1993) suggested that photic stimulation might be used as a disease probe. When Grady and associates (1997) presented subjects with a match-to-sample task in which task difficulty was systematically increased, there was a linearly increasing prefrontal cortex rCBF, whereas the rCBF in striate and extrastriate cortex was linearly decreased because the material required higher level processing than the passive task used in the Mentis et al. (1997) study. The passive task of just observing the photic stimulation activated more posterior areas and mental tasks of some degree of difficulty activated more anterior areas.

We reasoned that given this research, a technique that increases cerebral blood flow may at least partially remediate certain cognitive deficits if applied regularly over a period of time.[6] Siever (2000) speculates that the reduction of symptoms in people using AVS who suffer from ADHD, brain injury and aging is due to the increased blood flow and anaerobic conversion of glucose the AVS. The specific mechanisms that might be causing the type of clinical changes we've observed are discussed in detail in the next chapter of this book.

AVS WITH ELDERLY PATIENTS

In 1990, we began experimenting in our clinic with AVS in elderly patients. Initially, we chose 14Hz as the stimulation frequency because of research and clinical results relating to the activity in the narrow bands of 14Hz or 12–15Hz: Based on Giannitrapani's findings on the positive correlations between 13 and 14Hz single band power and I.Q. (1988), Sterman's work with epileptics (1996), Lubar's research with ADHD (Shouse & Lubar, 1979; Lubar et al., 1999), and numerous anecdotal reports, we concluded that the activity level in this frequency band is important for proper functioning of the brain (Budzynski, 1990). We completed several unpublished case and small group studies with this type of protocol, with significant success.

Several years later it was concluded that the use of AVS could enhance neurofeedback training even in the area of reversing age-related cognitive decline (Budzynski, 2000). We went on to design a pseudo-random AVS protocol, of the type described in the college student studies (previously mentioned), with the rationale of maximizing cerebral blood flow through constantly changing and randomized light/sound stimuli; in other words, minimizing adaptation effects. Combined with neurofeedback and other supplemental interventions, we had continued success with several patients who tried this intervention.

Recently, we decided to do a larger controlled study on cognitive enhancement in the elderly (Budzynski, Budzynski, & Tang, 2007). Thirty sessions of group AVS (20 minutes each) were given to an elderly group of individuals (N = 31).[7]

A waiting list control group took part in all the pre–post testing and they were offered the AVS training after they completed their part in the

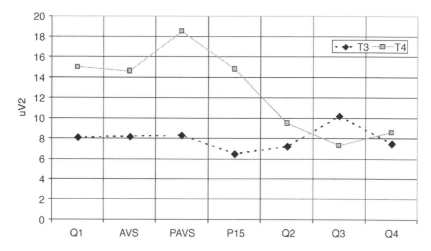

Figure 8.4 Percentage of seniors who increased, decreased, or remained the same after AVS.

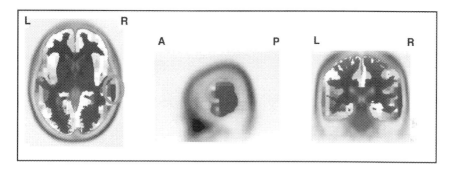

Figure 8.5 ARCD Study: Median post–pre Buschke and Microcog standard scores.

control group. The results, though not overwhelming, were encouraging in general. The pre–post POMs scale (Profile of Mood States) (Douglas, 1971/1981) revealed that approximately 50% of the experimental group showed decreased depression scores. The Symptoms of Stress Inventory (SOS) indicated that cognitive disorganization decreased. The Microcog test was also used to document other pre–post cognitive changes. A total of 31 participants were able to finish the training (this included former members of the C group who were offered and took the opportunity to get the AVS training). Figure 8.4 shows the percentage of participants who increased, decreased, or remained the same on each of the nine Microcog scales.

Figure 8.5 gives the post–pre Microcog results for the final E and C groups.

Several of the original members of each group were not included in this comparison because of development of or increasing severity of disease process or a major change in medication. The post–pre Reasoning difference between the groups might reflect the fact that the E group increased their speed of responding thus taking less time to make decisions. The Buschke test is a very telling short-term memory test on which the E group showed a slightly greater (improved)difference post–pre than the C group. The overall conclusion reached in the above study was that an AVS pseudo-random protocol appears to facilitate certain cognitive abilities and possibly improved mood, however, another AVS protocol may have been more effective.

AVS CASE STUDY ON ALZHEIMER'S DISEASE

In late November of 2000 we began a case study of a 57-year-old woman with a diagnosis of Alzheimer's Disease (AD). Both her mother and father had succumbed to the disease. KW agreed to participate in an initial study in which we would do a series of QEEGs (Q) to document the effects of AVS. A baseline Q was done, followed by 20 minutes of a pseudo-random AVS protocol, during which data for another Q was taken. A third Q was taken after the stimulation, and finally a fourth followed after a 15-minute rest period. The time course of all the Qs in this study was: Q1 baseline 10/3/00, Qs during, after, and post AVS in this first session; then Q2 (1/9/01) after 30 days of daily AVS; Q3 follow-up-1 (6/11/01); Q4 follow-up-2 (12/28/01).

Following the first session, KW was offered our clinic's 30-day group AVS training, and she decided to take it. It should be noted that KW showed significant improvements during her AVS training: She began walking alone to the training even though it was some blocks away. Also, her walking style changed from the flatfooted gait of the typical AD patient to a normal style. Friends noticed that she was speaking better, that is, finding words and annunciating more clearly. KW decided to use an AVS unit at home after she finished the training, however, we were later informed that she only used the unit intermittently and stopped using it altogether between Q2 and Q3.

KW'S QEEG ANALYSES

The analyses of KW's Qs were revealing. During the first session, the Q spectral analysis showed that the AVS resulted in decreased theta at T3 (left temporal) at the 15-minute post Q (Figure 8.6). However, in subsequent Qs theta at T3 did not differ much from baseline Q1. Theta at T4 (right temporal) was another story however. The values during the first session were unusually high, indicating that this right hemisphere area was quite probably more affected by the AD than the left. Interestingly, the theta at T4 decreased in Q2 and Q3 although KW had stopped using the home unit sometime after Q2. In Qs 2, 3, and 4 the level of theta at T4 was close to that at T3.

In October of 2001, some 10 months after the AVS training, KW underwent a SPECT scan, which revealed that the right hemisphere was more severely affected than the left by the AD. Did the AVS training decrease the slowing (theta) at T4? It would appear so from the data presented in Figure 8.6. Besides the usual quantification into various frequency band power/magnitudes at all 19 sites of the 10/20 International System, Lesley Sherlin, working with the Q data we had collected, used the new scanning technique called LORETA (Low-Resolution Electromagnetic Tomography; Pascual-Marqui, 1999) to determine deeper structural brain changes (Budzynski & Sherlin, 2002). Some of these images are shown in the previous figures.

LORETA data from several images can be subtracted to study the change that has taken place. Figure 8.7 shows the subtraction of Q1 from Q2 and the resultant image indicates a reduction in the theta band current density in both temporal areas, but primarily on the right side. This decrease was

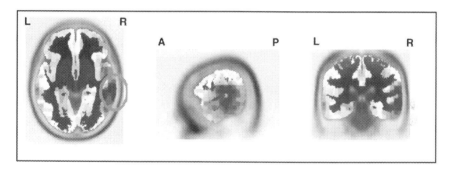

Figure 8.6 Theta power at T3 and T4 across Qs. Client: KW.

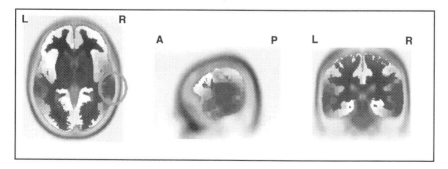

Figure 8.7 Q2–Q1 Theta. Theta decreased. Brodmann area 21, middle temporal gyrus, temporal lobe.

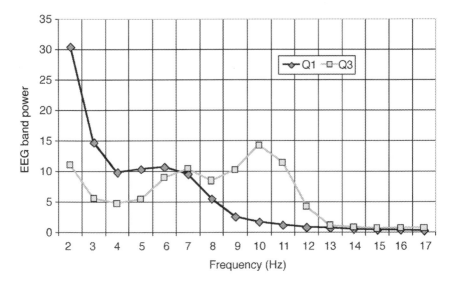

Figure 8.8   Q3–Q1 Theta. Theta decreased since Q1 and Q2. Brodmann area 21, middle temporal gyrus, temporal lobe.

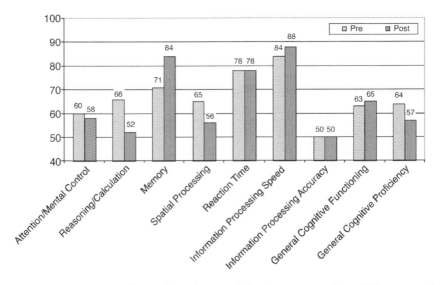

Figure 8.9   Q4–Q1 Theta. Theta decreased. Brodmann area 21, middle temporal gyrus, temporal lobe.

maintained in Q2 after the 30-day training, some 12 weeks later. The difference LORETA Q2-Q1 shows a decrease (blue) in theta in the right and left temporal areas and in the middle temporal gyrus after the 30-day training.

The next two images (Figures 8.8 and 8.9) show difference LORETAS comparing Q3 and Q4 with the Q1 baseline. In both cases the right temporal area indicates less theta than at baseline.

When the final Q4 was compared to baseline Q1, the temporal theta had decreased even more than at Q3. The pinkish color in Figure 8.8 indicates a slight elevation of theta in more medial areas. However, it is not apparent in Figure 8.9 when Q4 was compared to Q1.

Since AD seems to affect the temporal areas in the initial stages of AD, as evidenced by increasing theta, we have focused on the above images. There were a number of LORETAs made of other bands as well as theta, and all results are summarized next in Table 8.1.

The overall result was surprising in that the theta band power decreased from the baseline Q1 to the final Q4 and the delta band decreased at least to the time of Q3, even as the alpha and beta bands decreased.

These results are encouraging because theta and delta increases are among the earliest EEG changes seen in Alzheimer's Disease (Babiloni et al., 2007; Ponomareva, Korovaitseva, & Rogaev, 2007; Prichep, 2007). One can only wonder what would have happened if KW had been able to keep using the AVS regularly at home. One other EEG result is worth mentioning: As we noted earlier, the Peak Alpha Frequency (PAF) is an important indicator of brain health and performance (Nakano, Miyasaka, Ohtaka, & Ohomori, 1992; Matousek, Volavka, Roubicek, & Roth, 1967; Obrist, 1979). Most AD patients show very little alpha even in the eyes closed condition (Pricep et al., 1994) and such was true of KW in Q1. But Figure 8.10 shows that at least in the central parietal area (Pz) the Q3 analysis showed alpha peaking at 10Hz, whereas the Q1 showed only a slight increase at 6Hz. Note also that the slow frequency 2–6Hz band power is decreased in Q3. Finally, KW's pre–post 30-day AVS training Microcog scores are shown in Figure 8.11.

In keeping with her subjective report of an increased ability to multi-task and remember where she put things, her Memory score showed the greatest improvement of all 9 scales. Taking this in sum, the AVS training did appear to produce some positive changes in KW's brain.

Table 8.1   Changes Compared to Q1

	Q2	Q3	Q4	Overall
Delta	*Declined*	*Improved*	*Declined*	*Mixed*
Theta	*Improved*	*Improved*	*Improved*	*Improved*
Alpha	*Declined*	*Declined*	*Declined*	*Declined*
Beta1	*Declined*	*Declined*	*Declined*	*Declined*
Beta2	*Declined*	*Declined*	*Declined*	*Declined*

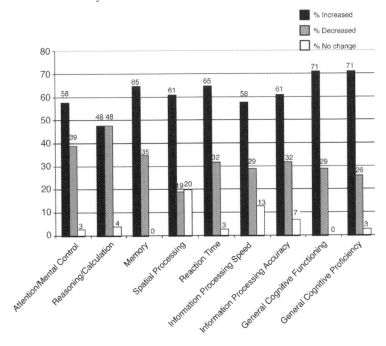

Figure 8.10   Frequency spectrum at Pz in Q1 and Q3. Subject: KW.

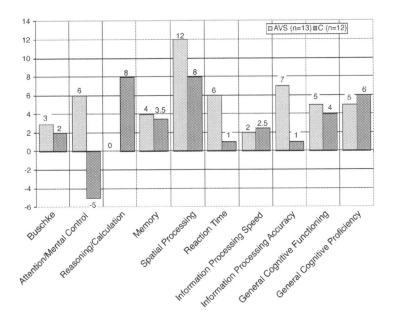

Figure 8.11   Pre-post session AVS training—Microcog standard scores. KW-AD diagnosis..

TENTATIVE CONCLUSIONS ABOUT AVS AND ALZHEIMER'S

1. AVS would seem to produce, at least temporarily, some enhancement of memory ability even in the case of a moderately severe AD patient.
2. AVS seems to restore, at least temporarily, some degree of spatial ability. For example, KW noted, as a result of the training, she was able to accurately find her way around a several block radius including the distance from her home to the site of the AVS training.
3. Her walking style improved from the shuffling, flatfooted stride of many AD patients to a cautious normal gait.
4. She reported that the cognitive fog lifted after her training.
5. EEG changes included decreases in the delta band in the frontal, temporal, and parietal areas. These lasted at least 15 minutes after stimulation, and in fact, the Q3 delta was reduced compared to Q1.
6. The theta EEG power at T4 was initially significantly increased over that at T3 however, after the AVS training (and some home AVS use), the theta at T4 came down to the lower level shown at T3.
7. Although the alpha/theta ratio decreases dramatically in most AD patients, in the case of KW her Q3 values actually increased in posterior areas. Her T4 (right temporal) showed an increasing slope of alpha/theta ratio across Qs even out to Q4.
8. Peak alpha frequency (PAF) was increased in the parietal area with continued use of the home AVS up to Q3.
9. Finally, the Microcog Reasoning/Calculation scale seemed to be lower in the post score of KW as well as in the larger group of elderly people used in the previous study (presented earlier). Perhaps this variable will need to be watched carefully in future AVS applications, especially with the elderly.

STROKE AND PHOTIC STIMULATION

We were able to test the effects of photic stimulation (PS) on the brain of an aphasic individual (Rozelle & Budzynski, 1995). JY had suffered a massive left hemisphere stroke more than 6 months before. As part of the treatment we used an early EEG Driven Stimulation (EDS) prototype (Ochs & Berman, 1994; Larsen, 2006)[8]. An LED array goggle eyepiece incorporated bright visual stimulation with the frequency driven by the subject's EEG. The actual LED frequency was flashed at intervals of some percentage above and at times below the EEG dominant frequency at F7 or the left frontal area. The time spent at any one stimulating frequency could be varied. A second part of the treatment was neurofeedback based on activity at F7. The client himself requested a return to the EDS protocol for the final part of his training. The client's recovery was so successful that he wrote a book, *Up From the Ashes: There is Life After a Stroke,* (Young, 1995) and spent the next few years offering workshops on successful stroke recovery.

A FINAL WORD

Audio-visual stimulation will continue to be an important part of our therapy protocols and we will no doubt be applying cautiously a number of frequency, LED color, and sound variations in the clinic. Increasing use of fMRI, MEG, and the new high resolution SPECT scanners will enable researchers to delineate very specific areas activated or suppressed by AVS. It is also quite probable that as AVS protocols are compared at conferences and through Internet communication they will become increasingly more selective and effective. A national protocol and treatment database is badly needed to encourage standardization of treatments, both to encourage the safe use of AVS and to make systematic research in this field more viable and practical.

NOTES

1. See Chapters 1 and 9 in this volume for literature reviews on AVS.
2. As with PAF, the A3/A1 ratio tends to decrease with age, brain injury, and dementia (Matousek et al., 1967; Nakano et al., 1992; Kuskowski, Mortimer, Morley, Malone, & Okaya, 1993; Prichep et al., 1994).
3. See Chapters 1, 7, and 9.
4. See mindbyte.net.
5. A common observation of those who use AVS is that a sudden external noise seems to momentarily heighten the brightness of the photic stimulation. This synesthesia may also manifest when music is combined with photic stimulation. Robert Austin of Synetic Systems incorporates a technique called "Polysynch" in which the first few digitally encoded bits on his music cassettes or CDs program his AVS units such that the resulting light/sound (music) program is perfectly coordinated with the musical piece to give a dramatic effect to the session. Perhaps the synesthesia works both ways with the photic stimulation driving audio enhancements and the audio variations driving changes in the perceived visual stimulation. It is our observation that the synesthesia effects seem to occur more often when the light or sound changes are unexpected.
6. Certain parameters of the EEG tend to correlate with the cerebral profusion, at least in the neocortex (Fried, 1993), thus, an area of hypoperfusion will tend to be mirrored by the increase of theta band (4–8Hz) power in the EEG on the scalp surface in that location.
7. Comptronics, Inc. donated an AVS training system consisting of a master AVS unit and 10 satellite boxes driven off the master that allowed each subject to independently adjust light intensity and sound volume in their own goggles and headphones.
8. See Chapter 9 for more on this.

REFERENCES

Alexander, G. E., Prohovnik, I., Stem, Y., & Mayeux, R. (1994). WAIS-R subtest profile and cortical perfusion in Alzheimer's Disease. *Brain and Cognition, 2*(4), 24–43.

Anderson, D. J. (1989). The treatment of migraine with variable frequency photic stimulation. *Headache, 29,* 154–155.

Anoukhin, A., & Vogel, F. (1996). EEG alpha rhythm frequency and intelligence in normal individuals. *Intelligence, 23,* 1–14.

Babiloni, C., Cassetta, E., Binetti, G., Tombini, M., Del Percio, C., Ferreri, F., . . . Rossini, P. M. (2007). Resting EEG sources correlate with attentional span in mild cognitive impairment and Alzheimer's disease. *European Journal of Neuroscience, 25*(12), 3742–3757.

Budzynski, T. H. (1990). *Single and double Hz band EEG results in normals and dysfunctional individuals.* Futurehealth Neurofeedback Conference. Key West, FL.

Budzynski, T. H. (1991a). *Clinical considerations of light/sound.* Synetic Systems. Seattle, WA.

Budzynski, T. H. (1991b). *Selected research on light/sound.* Synetic Systems, Seattle WA.

Budzynski, T. H. (2000). Reversing age-related cognitive decline: Use of neurofeedback and audio-visual stimulation. *Biofeedback, 28,* 19–21.

Budzynski, T., Budzynski, H., & Tang, H. Y. (2007). Brain brightening: Restoring the aging mind. In J. R. Evans (Ed.), *Handbook of neurofeedback: Dynamics and clinical applications.* New York: Hayworth Press, 231–265.

Budzynski, T., Jordy, J., Kogan Budzynski, H., Tang, J., & Claypoole, K. (1999). Academic performance enhancement with photic stimulation and EDR feedback. *Journal of Neurotherapy, 3,* 11–21.

Budzynski, T., & Sherlin, L. (2002). *Short and long-term AVS (audio-visual stimulation) effects in an Alzheimer's patient as documented by QEEG and LORETA.* Presented at the Futurehealth Winter Brain Meeting. Palm Springs, CA.

Budzynski, T. H., & Stoyva, J. (1984). Biofeedback methods in the treatment of anxiety and stress. In R. Woolfolk & P. Lehrer (Eds.), *Principle and practice of stress management.* New York: The Guilford Press, 263–300.

Budzynski, T. H., & Tang, J. (1998). *Biolight effects on the EEG.* SynchroMed Report. Seattle, WA.

Celsis, P., Agniel, A., Cardebat, D., Demonet, J. F., Ousett, P. J., & Puel, M. (1997). Age related cognitive decline: A clinical entity? A longitudinal study of cerebral blood flow and memory performance. *Journal of Neurology, Neurosurgery, and Psychiatry, 62,* 601–608.

Carter, J., & Russell, H. (1993). A pilot investigation of auditory and visual entrainment of brainwave activity in learning disabled boys. *Texas Researcher: Journal of Texas Center for Educational Research, 4,* 65–73.

Doppelmayr, M., Klimesch, W., Hodlmoser, K., Sauseng, P., & Gruber, W. (2005). Intelligence related upper alpha desynchronization in a semantic memory task. *Brain Research Bulletin, 66,* 171–177.

Doppelmayr, M., Klimesch, W., Sauseng, P., Hodlmoser, K., Stadler, W., & Hanslmayr, S. (2005). Intelligence related differences in EEG-bandpower. *Neuroscience Letters, 381,* 309–313.

Douglas, M. (1971/1981). *Profile of mood states: Manual.* San Diego: Educational and Industrial Testing Service.

Fox, P., & Raichle, M. (1985). Stimulus rate determines regional blood flow in striate cortex. *Annals of Neurology, 17,* 303–305.

Fox, P., Raichle, M., Mintun, M., & Dence, C. (1988). Nonoxidative glucose consumption during focal physiologic neural activity. *Science, 241,* 462–464.

Fried, R. (1993). What is theta? *Biofeedback and Self-Regulation, 18,* 53–58.

Giannitrapani, D. (1969). EEG average frequency and intelligence. *EEG and Clinical Neurophysiology, 27,* 480–486.

Giannitrapani, D. (1988). The role of 13-Hz activity in mentation. In D. Giannitrapani & L. Murri (Eds.), *The EEG of mental activities* (pp. 149–152). New York: Karger.

Grady, C. L., Horwitz, B., Pietrini, P., Mentis, M. J., Ungerleider, L. G., Rapoport, S. I., & Haxby, J. V. (1997). Effect of task difficulty on cerebral blood flow during perceptual matching of faces. *Human Brain Mapping, 4,* 227–239.

Gur, R. C., Gur, R. E., Obrist, W. D., Skolnick, B. E., & Reivich, M. (1987). Age and regional cerebral blood flow at rest and during cognitive activity. *Archives of General Psychiatry, 44*, 617–621.

Heiss, W. D., Pawlik, G., Holthoff, V., Kessler, J., & Szelies, B. (1992). PET correlates of normal and impaired memory functions. *Cerebrovascular and Brain Metabolism Reviews, 4*, 1–27.

Jausovec, N. (1996). Differences in EEG alpha activity related to giftedness. *Intelligence, 23*, 159–173.

Klimesch, W., Doppelmayr, M., Pachinger, T., & Ripper, B. (1997). Brain oscillations and human memory: EEG correlates in the upper alpha and theta band. *Neuroscience Letters, 238*, 9–12.

Klimesch, W., Schack, B., & Sauseng, P. (2005). The functional significance of theta and upper alpha oscillations. *Experimental Psychology, 52*, 99–108.

Kuskowski, M., Mortimer, J., Morley, G., Malone, S., & Okaya, A. (1993). Rate of cognitive decline in Alzheimer's disease associated with EEG alpha power. *Biological Psychiatry, 33*(8–9), 659–662.

Larsen, S. (2006). *The healing power of neurofeedback: The revolutionary LENS technique for restoring optimal brain function.* Rochester, VT: Healing Arts Press.

Lubar, J. and Lubar, J. (1999). Neurofeedback assessment and treatment for attention deficit hyperactivity disorder in Evans, J. and Abarbanel, A. (Eds.) *Quantitative EEG and Neurofeedback*, San Diego, CA, pp. 103–146.

Matousek, E., Volavka, J., Roubicek, J., & Roth, Z. (1967). EEG frequency analysis related to age in normal adults. *Electroencephalography and Clinical Neurophysiology, 23*, 162–167.

Melamed, E., Lavy, S., Bentin, S., Cooper, G., & Rinot, Y. (1980). Reduction in regional cerebral blood flow during normal aging in man. *Stroke, 11*, 31–35.

Mentis, M., Alexander, G., Grady, C., Horwitz, B., Krasuski, J., Pietrini, P., . . . Rapoport, S. (1997). Frequency variation of a pattern-flash visual stimulus during PET differentially activates brain from the striate through frontal cortex. *Neuroimage, 5*, 116–128.

Meyer, J. S., Terayama, Y., & Takashima, S. (1993). Cerebral circulation in the elderly. *Cerebrovascular and Brain Metabolism Reviews, 5*, 122–146.

Mints, A.Y., Litinvenko, A. A., & Bachinskaya, N. Y. (1987–1988). Cerebral circulation and certain parameters of the functional state of the brain in the process of aging. *Soviet Neurology and Psychiatry*, Winter–Spring.

Nagahama, Y., Fukuyama, H., Yamauchi, H., Katsumi, Y., Magata, Y., Shibasaki, H., & Kimura, J. (1997). Age-related changes in cerebral blood flow activation during a Card Sorting Test. *Experimental Brain Research, 114*, 571–577.

Nakano, T., Miyasaka, M., Ohtaka, T., & Ohomori, L. (1992). Longitudinal changes in computerized EEG and mental functions of the aged: A nine-year follow-up study. *International Psychogeriatrics, 41*, 9–23.

Ochs, L., & Berman, M. (1994). *EDS: Background and operation.* Walnut Creek, CA: Flexyx, LLC.

Obrist, W. O. (1979). Electroencephalographic changes in normal aging and dementia. *Brain Function in Old Age*, pp. 102–111.

Pascal-Marqui, R. D., Lehman, D., Koenig, T. et al. (1999). Low resolution brain electromagnetic tomography (LORETA) functional imaging in acute neuroleptic-naïve first episode productive Schizophrenia, *Psychiatry Res.* 90, 169–179.

Pascal-Marqui, R. D., Michel, C. M., & Lehmann, D. (1994). Low resolution electromagnetic tomography: A new method for localizing electrical activity in the brain. *International Journal of Psychophysiology, 18*, 49–65.

Peterson, R., Smith, G., Kokmen, E., Ivnid, R., & Tangalos, E. (1992). Memory function in normal aging. *Neurology, 42*, 396–401.

Ponomareva, N. V., Korovaitseva, G. I., & Rogaev, E. I. (2007). EEG alterations in non-demented individuals related to apolipoprotein E genotype and to risk of Alzheimer disease. *Neurobiology Aging*, February 9 [Epub ahead of print: PMID: 17293007].

Pricep, L., John, E., Ferris, S., Reisberg, B., Almas, M., Alper, K., & Cancro, R. (1994). Quantitative EEG correlates of cognitive deterioration in the elderly. *Neurobiology of Aging*, 15(1), 85–90.

Prichep, L. S. (2007). Quantitative EEG and electromagnetic brain imaging in aging and in the evolution of dementia. *Annals of the New York Academy of Sciences*, 1097, 156–167.

Rapoport, S. I., & Grady, C. L. (1993). Parametric in vivo brain imaging during activation to examine pathological mechanisms of functional failure in Alzheimer disease. *International Journal of Neuroscience*, 70, 39–56.

Rozelle, G. R., & Budzynski, T. H. (1995). Neurotherapy for stroke rehabilitation: A single case study. *Biofeedback and Self-Regulation*, 20, 211–228.

Russell, H. L. (1997). Intellectual functioning, auditory and photic stimulation and changes in functioning in children and adults. *Biofeedback*, 25, 16–24.

Sappey-Mariner, et al. (1992). Effect of photic stimulation on human visual cortex lactate and phosphates using 1H and 31P Magnetic Resonance Spectroscopy. *Journal of Cerebral Blood Flow and Metabolism*, 12, 584–592.

Sauseng, P., Klimesch, W., Schabus, M., & Doppelmayr, M. (2005). Frontoparietal EEG coherence in theta and upper alpha reflect central executive functions of working memory. *International Journal of Psychophysiology*, 57, 97–103.

Shouse, M. N., & Lubar, J. F. (1979). Operant conditioning of EEG rhythms and ritalin in the treatment of hyperkinesis. *Biofeedback Self-Regulation*, 4(4), 299–312.

Siever, D. (2003a). Audio-visual entrainment: 1. History and physiological mechanisms. *Biofeedback*, 31(2), 21–27.

Siever, D. (2003b). Audio-visual entrainment: II. Dental studies. *Biofeedback*, 31(3), 29–32.

Siever, D. (2003c). Applying audio-visual entrainment technology for attention and learning Part III. *Biofeedback*, 31(4), 24–29.

Siever, D. (2005). The application of audio-visual entrainment for the treatment of seniors issues: Part 1. *Biofeedback*, 33, 109–113.

Solomon, G. D. (1985). Slow wave photic stimulation in the treatment of headache a preliminary study. *Headache*, 25, 444–446.

Sterman, M. B. (1996). Physiological origins and functional correlates of EEG rhythmic activities: Implications for self-regulation. *Biofeedback Self-Regulation*, 21(1), 3–33.

Vogt, F., Klimesch, W., & Doppelmayr, M. (1998). High-frequency components in the alpha band and memory performance. *Journal of Clinical Neurophysiology*, 15, 167–172.

Waldemar, G. (1995). Functional brain imaging with SPECT in normal aging and dementia. *Cerebrovascular and Brain Metabolism Reviews*, 7, 89–130.

Wszolek, Z. K., Herkes, G. K., Lagerlund, T. D., & Kokmen, E. (1992). Comparison of EEG background frequency analysis, psychologic test scores, short test of mental status, and quantitative SPECT in dementia. *Journal of Geriatric Psychiatry and Neurology*, 5, 22–30.

Wu, X., & Liu, X. Q. (1995). Study of the alpha frequency band of healthy in quantitative EEG. *Clinical Electroencephalography*, 26, 131–136.

Wyper, D. J. (1993). Functional neuroimaging with single photon emission computed tomography (SPECT). *Cerebrovascular and Brain Metabolism Reviews*, 5, 199–217.

Young, J. (1995). *Up from the ashes: There is life after a stroke*. Pensacola, FL: The Inner Path.

9 Rhythmic Sensory Stimulation of the Brain

The Possible Use of Inexpensive Sensory Stimulation Technologies to Improve IQ Test Scores and Behavior

Harold Russell and Gabe Turow

OVERVIEW

It has long been accepted that specific kinds of increases in physical activity can result in specific kinds of long lasting increases in physical functioning or abilities. There is increasing scientific evidence that specific kinds of increases in brain or neuronal activity can result in long-lasting increases in specific kinds of brain functioning or abilities.

The purpose of this chapter is to explore the hypothesis that when two specific forms of rhythmic sensory stimulation of the brain are combined— the extended use of repetitive EEG-Driven Light and Sound Stimulation (rEDLSS) and the extended listening to, learning, practicing, and playing of specific music—it can result in long-lasting increased cognitive abilities in children, as measured by increases in IQ test scores.

The underlying concept (we will argue through research evidence) is that both of these two forms of stimulation can induce increases in the amount of synchronous "firing" of hundreds of millions of brain cells. Long-term increases in the amount of "firing" (neuronal activation) can, in turn, result in increases in the complexity, size, and efficiency of the actual physical structure of the brain. Changes in form can then allow changes in functioning that can be measured: by increases or changes in patterns of EEG activity, as changes in regional cerebral blood flow (rCBF) or changes in brain chemistry. Behavioral level changes, such as improvements in working memory, may occur as indicators of increased brain growth and development in children. Behavioral changes can act as indicators of recovery from trauma or of improvement in people with age-related decreases in brain functioning.

Recent neuroplasticity research continues to confirm that the brain retains its ability, from infancy to old age, to modify its physical structure and increase its functioning in response to changes in its ongoing environment.

Evidence is presented here that increases in the levels of brain activity can result in physical changes in brain microstructure, such as increases in the number and efficiency of synapses (synaptogenesis), or changes in brain chemistry, for example, increases in brain-derived neurotrophic factor (BDNF) that increase the brain's ability to adapt to and respond to changes in, or to increasing demands from, the brain's environment. In light of this, the indications that rEDLSS and music may share a common mechanism of action and may have similar and positive effects on children's abilities to learn are explored in depth. There is a definite possibility that a synergistic interaction exists between these two stimulation modalities. Their combined use could reasonably result in greater increases in the levels of brain activity than would be observed if they were used singly or in sequence. The data presented here suggests that a synthesis of these two forms of stimulation could be applied to the treatment of learning disabilities and attention deficit disorders (LD/ADD/ADHD). If effective, this modality could potentially be extremely inexpensive to administer to children and adults. There is already almost universal access to music and stereo systems, and the low cost of rEDLSS could make this combination available to individuals of all socioeconomic levels.

There are many different forms of brain stimulation currently being investigated as a means of stimulating increases in the activity of millions of brain cells to induce positive brain changes. Examples are electrical deep-brain stimulation (DBS) from surgically implanted electrodes, cranial electrical stimulation (CES), and repetitive transcranial magnetic stimulation (rTMS). However, a discussion of these other methods and their uses is beyond the scope of this chapter.

PART I. rEDLSS AND ATTENTION DEFICIT DISORDER

What is rEDLSS?

rEDLSS is a technology that was developed and field-tested over a 3-year period with funding from a U.S. Department of Education/SBIR award as a potential treatment for children with learning disabilities and attention deficit disorder problems. rEDLSS uses combined pulses of auditory and visual stimuli to repetitively activate hundreds of millions of brain cells in the auditory and visual areas of the brain. The frequency of the incoming stimulation is individually controlled by the constantly varying dominant frequency of each person's brainwave (EEG) activity. Close matching of the incoming stimuli to ongoing brainwave activity has been shown to result in increasingly large areas of the brain matching their activity to the constantly varying frequencies of the incoming stimuli (see Chapters 1, 2, 5, 7, 8, this volume). The rEDLSS allows each person's EEG activity to determine the kind and amount of stimulation that flows into their brain—as the activity changes in the brain, the rEDLSS responds with slightly different stimulation. There is entrainment between the rEDLSS unit and the user: The rEDLSS is affecting the user's rhythms, which are then affecting the setup (the computer responds by changing the light and sound pattern's frequency), which then affects the user, and so on.

In practice, light stimulation is presented via glasses fitted with light emitting diodes (LEDs) and the auditory stimulation is played through normal headphones. Pulsed monaural sine tones and binaural beat stimuli are used as the auditory component of the stimulation (see Chapter 7 for a full explanation of binaural beats. Also see Lane, Kasian, Owens, & Marsh, 1998). When rEDLSS treatment is used, brainwave (EEG) activity is continuously measured and analyzed and the results are used to dynamically adjust the patterns of audiovisual stimulation towards patient- and pathology-determined activation targets.

How is rEDLSS Used, and What is the Basis for Its Efficacy?

Research has shown an association between various neurological disorders, including Alzheimer's, Parkinson's, and Attention Deficit Disorders. Although these three disorders are considered discrete disease entities, they all show differing and anomalous or atypical cerebral blood flow (CBF) patterns, reflecting (at least in part) differing and anomalous or atypical patterns of brain electrical activity (Mori, 2002; Lou et al., 2004; Ors et al., 2005; Sigi-Hale, Bookheimer, McGough, Phillips, & McCracken, 2007). A variety of abnormalities in brain chemistry may be observed when blood flow in and to the region of activity is decreased as a result of diminished electrical activity or a downward shift in EEG frequencies.

A recent animal study from Brown, Davies, and Randall (2007, p. 1460) suggests: "convergent afferent synaptic activity can alter the precise temporal arrangement of neuronal network activity." A somewhat similar suggestion, in another animal study, is proposed by Holtzman at Cambridge (2006, p. 491): "cerebellar cortical activity can be powerfully modulated by the general level of peripheral afferent [incoming stimuli] activation from much of the body."

The use of massive amounts of peripheral afferent stimulation during a brief time span (2 to 3 weeks of intensive treatment) has been reported by Taub and his collaborators to result in marked recovery of functioning in the impaired limb in both child and adult stroke patients, independent of the time post-stroke (see review by Taub et al., 2007; Wolf et al., 2010). The afferent stimuli are generated by forced use of the impaired extremity while the unimpaired limb is constrained (a treatment called Constraint Induced Movement Therapy).

Stimulation-induced increases in neural activation may someday be shown to have a direct influence on several of the fundamental causes of neurological disorders, such as the reduced cerebral blood flow (hypoperfusion) observed in studies of patients with dementias (Lewy bodies, Parkinson's and Alzheimer's; e.g., Brockhuis et al., 2006; Mito et al., 2005; Mazza, Marano, Traversi, Bria, & Mazza, 2010).

Studies suggest that increased blood flow also plays an important role in the stimulation of neuronal plasticity, that is, the ability of the brain to reorganize itself in response to its ongoing experience and to trauma (for detailed reviews of use-dependent neuronal plasticity, synaptogenesis, and neurogenesis, see Johansson 2000, 2003, 2004, 2006, 2007, 2010; Wan & Schlaug, 2010; Skoe & Kraus, 2010). Independent but scientifically related reports (Kilgard, Panda, Engineer, & Moucha, 2002; Pleger et al., 2003; Kolb, 2003; Marshall, 2007) present strong support for the use of sensory stimulation to induce reorganization or "re-wiring" of the cortex. Zito and Svoboda (2002, p. 1015) at Cold Spring Harbor Laboratory, explain that: "the adult cortex generates new synapses in response to sensory activity and these structural changes can occur rapidly, within 24 hours of sensory stimulation."

A review by Miles (2005) and a report of later work by McDonnell et al. (2007) agree with these formulations: "The normal human cortex can be made to reorganize by repeated stimulation of proprioceptive inputs" (2005, p. 128) and "Reorganization of the human motor cortex can be induced by specific patterns of peripheral afferent stimulation" (2007, p. 435).

Kilgard and Merzenich (2002) summarize the findings from animal research that manipulating sensory experience results in systematic changes in the functional organization of the adult primary auditory cortex. A variety of studies involving high levels of sensory inputs flowing into the brain (afferent stimulation) from enriched environments (which evoke increases in brain or neuronal activity) have reported increased brain functioning and increased brain complexity in animals (Diamond, 1988, 2001; Rosenzwieg & Bennett, 1996; Rosenzwieg, 2003).

Additionally, it appears that increasing the levels of neuronal electrical activity and blood flow in areas of delayed maturation (associated with ADHD) or damaged areas (stroke, trauma, etc.) can up-regulate the production of neurotrophins, which enhance the ability of the brain to re-organize itself (Patz & Wahle, 2004). Research results also suggests that the therapeutic effects of repeated and prolonged neural activation may result in a reversal of some of the more troubling symptoms of some neurological disorders or perhaps a slowing of disease progress in other disorders (see Chapters 6, 8).

Intermittent photic stimulation (IPS) is widely considered to be one of the most powerful techniques available for stimulating neural activity (Lazarev, Simpson, Schubsky, & DeAzevedo, 2001). An indication of its potential comes from recent research reports that have documented some recovery of vision in patients with partial cortical blindness. Repetitive and prolonged tachistoscopic (a form of intermittent photic) stimulation of their visual cortex was used during several months of treatment (Pleger et al., 2003; Widdig, Pleger, Rommel, Malin, & Tegenthoff, 2003; Marshall et al., 2007). Widdig and colleagues write of one of their patients that:

[this] statistically significant improvement of different visual functions and a reoccurrence of visual abilities important in daily life did not

only signify a greater degree of independence but, above all, a considerable increase in his quality of life. (2003, p. 235)

Rhythmic auditory stimulation, on the other hand, activates a smaller but mostly differing set of neural structures than IPS (Pastor et al., 2002; Pastor, Artieda, Arbizu, Valencia, & Masdeu, 2003) and similarly has clinical value regarding the reorganization of the cortex and treatment of neurological disorders (also see Chapter 6).

The combined use of these two sensory modalities results in a noninvasive stimulation method known as repetitive EEG-Driven Light and Sound Stimulation (rEDLSS), which utilizes repetitive rhythmic (intermittent) photic and auditory stimulation to induce the controlled and synchronous activation of hundreds of millions of brain cells.

It is important to understand that the rEDLSS provides approximately 600–900 auditory and visual pulses per minute (12,000–18,000 paired stimuli per 20-minute session for 40 sessions). Most subjects reported finding the stimulation enjoyable and not at all overwhelming (Carter & Russell, 1995). As we will discuss in detail in Part II of this chapter, repetitive audiovisual stimulation has previously been reported to increase cerebral blood flow and oxygen metabolism (Yamauchi, Okazawa, Kishibe, Sugimoto, & Takahashi, 2002), influence electrocortical activity and autonomic reactivity (Brauchli, Michel, & Zeier, 1995), and modulate other aspects of cellular chemistry.

The U.S. Department of Education/SBIR funded a $230,000, 3-year controlled study on the cognitive and behavioral effects of rEDLSS on over 120 LD/ADD/ADHD children (Carter & Russell, 1993, 1994, 1995; Russell, 1996). Russell collaborated with John Carter, a professor in the School of Education Studies at the University of Houston, Clear Lake. The experiments, in addition to two pilot studies on rEDLSS and ADHD (Carter & Russell, 1993), consistently demonstrated significant and lasting improvements in cognition and behavior in children with attention deficit/hyperactivity disorder (ADHD). The results of the U.S. Department of Education/SBIR study showed statistically significant increases in IQ test scores (9.7) and behavioral gains in the experimental group of children over an 8-week, 40-session period of treatment.

The experimental group IQ test scores increased by 4.2 points during the first 20 sessions. A 5.5-point increase was observed during the second 20 sessions, representing approximately a 30% larger gain. The reasons for the larger gains during the second 20 sessions are as yet unclear although it can be speculated that changes in brain microstructure during the first 20 sessions may have contributed to the larger gains in the second 20 sessions.

These gains were maintained on a 16-month follow-up, strongly suggesting that improvements, once made, are maintained and may even increase if the gains are used daily in learning activities in the classroom. This research is presented in more detail later in this chapter.

The diversity of application studies in this area (also see Chapter 8) suggests that rEDLSS may have the potential to be a platform technology for the treatment of some neurological disorders. *It may well be particularly worthwhile to explore its use with those disorders characterized by decreased electrical activity and decreased cerebral blood flow as a result of developmental delays, trauma, or the effects of normal aging.*

How Could rEDLSS Work With Music-Listening/Playing?

Acquisition of musical skills and the effects of music learning on the brain has been a focus of plasticity research, which complements a long-held folk belief that stimulation of the brain by studying, learning, practicing, and listening to music improves the functioning of the brain.

There is a very extensive body of scientific literature documenting the short and long-term effects of music on the development, structure and functioning of the brain from infancy throughout the life span. This is considered to be evidence of activity-based or experience-based brain plasticity (Rauscher, 2001; Trainor, Shahin, & Roberts, 2003; Pantev, 2003). Typical comments are those made by Johansson (2004, p. 231; Johansson, 2010) who states: "Early musical training has lasting effects in shaping the brain." Currently, scientific investigations of this long-held folk belief in the beneficial effects of music on brain functioning are being conducted at several universities, for example, Stanford (Sridharan, Levitin, Chafe, Berger, & Menon, 2007), McGill (Levitin, 2005; Zatorre, Chen, & Penhune, 2007; Kim & Zatorre, 2010; Peretz et al., 2009), Harvard (Schlaug, Norton, Overy, & Winner, 2005; Wan & Schlaug, 2010), Colorado (Thaut, 2005; Thaut et al., 2009), and many others. Researchers have presented strong evidence based on brain imaging that both the structure and functioning of the brain are changed or improved by the rhythmic sensory stimulation it receives from music. Current evidence from many of these studies strongly suggests that the extent of the changes observed is proportional to the amount of musical stimulation experienced (although the time frame for change is often cited in terms of being hundreds or thousands of hours).

Many people may think of music as providing stimulation only to auditory areas of the brain. The rhythmic sensory stimulation of the brain generated by musical experience is actually highly complex. As Zatorre (2003, 2007) and Schlaug have observed (2005), the acquiring of musical proficiency involves the learning, practice, and continuous integration of many different kinds of complex skills. Because of this, music acquisition involves a large cognitive component. In this light, music could be properly described as rhythmic sensory-cognitive stimulation, given "new findings that music can stimulate complex cognitive, affective, and sensorimotor processes in the brain, which can then be generalized and transferred to nonmusical therapeutic purposes" (Thaut, 2005, p. 303).

Two related studies (Rauscher et al., 1997; Graziano, Peterson, Shaw, 1999) have explored the effects of music on spatial-temporal (ST) reasoning, which involves maintaining and transforming mental images in the absence of a physical model and is required for higher brain functions such as chess, mathematics, and engineering (1997, p. 2). Rauscher reported that musical training causes long-term enhancement of preschool children's spatial-temporal reasoning. Graziano reported that a combination of music training (keyboard training) and spatial-temporal training resulted in experimental group second grade children scoring significantly higher on the learning of proportional math and fractions than control group children. Also, recently, musical training has been reported to increase the amount of simultaneous or synchronous higher frequency brainwave activity (gamma-band coherence) involved in a faster and more accurate integration or synthesis of information from different parts of the brain (Thaut, Peterson, & McIntosh, 2005; Peterson & Thaut, 2007). In regard to the effect that musical training may have on memory, Groussard et al. (2010, p. 14) write: "Our findings support the idea that musical training may be associated with the development of specific memory abilities that could contribute to a greater cognitive reserve, which could reduce age-related decline in memory."

Brain imaging studies using fMRI (Gaser & Schlaug, 2003), comparing musicians and non-musicians, have shown changes in multiple areas in addition to the auditory. These changes are positively correlated with the amount of exposure to the musical stimuli. In the opinion of Zatorre at McGill University (2003, 2005, 2007): "Music performance is one of the most complex and demanding cognitive challenges that the human mind can undertake" (2007, p. 547). Schlaug at Harvard (2005, p. 219) explains that: "when functional and structural differences are found between the brains of matched musicians and non-musician controls, it is because musicians acquire and continuously practice a variety of complex motor, auditory, and multimodal skills (e.g., translating visually perceived musical symbols into motor commands while simultaneously monitoring instrumental output and receiving multisensory feedback)."

Schlaug comments further: "Research has also demonstrated that music training in children results in long-term enhancement of visual-spatial, verbal, and mathematical performance. However, the neural bases of such enhancements are as yet unknown" (2005, p. 219). "Though the pathways and mechanisms behind these increases in cognitive performance are not well understood, research has indicated that musicians' brains differ from those of non-musicians in important and measurable ways and in several anatomically distinct brain regions. This is thought to make it more likely that the differences observed are adaptations to long-term musical practice and less likely that the differences are innate, that is, genetic" (Gaser & Schlaug, 2003). The differences appear to increase in direct proportion to the years of brain stimulation arising from musical experience (training, study, and practice), that is, childhood musical training continued into adulthood appears to have a major influence on brain growth and development throughout the life span (Gaser & Schlaug, 2003; Schellenberg, 2007; Wan & Schlaug, 2010).

Looking at the research as a whole, it seems likely that music and rEDLSS could work together to stimulate many areas of the brain at the same time. The stimulation generated by the rEDLSS is primarily focused on stimuli to auditory and visual areas, whereas music stimulation is more diffuse and targets many areas of the brain simultaneously. The amount of auditory, visual, and motor stimuli generated by musical experience has not been shown to be adequate to produce the kinds of rapid changes observed after only 800 minutes (40, 20-minute sessions, a typical treatment course) of the more narrowly focused auditory and visual stimuli generated by the rEDLSS. There is a distinct possibility that the amount of time required for musically induced changes to occur could be drastically reduced if the large increases in auditory and visual stimuli inputs generated by the rEDLSS could be combined with or added to the more diffuse stimulation generated by music, either sequentially or concurrently. In addition, it is possible that the rapidity of learning musical skills (and the effects of learning them) could be increased significantly.

More intelligent children tend to learn many other skills more quickly than less intelligent children. If the fairly brief use of rEDLSS (800 minutes) over a short period of time (8 weeks) results in higher IQ tests scores (Russell & Carter, 1996), then there is reason to suspect that some of the same brain changes that enable children to score higher on IQ tests after rEDLSS training may be some of the same factors that could enable them to learn the highly complex skills involved in playing music after rEDLSS training. This is an easily testable hypothesis.

Studies by Yamamoto and colleagues (2004) as well as by Zangeneh-pour and Zatorre (2010) have begun to explore the issue of combining different forms of stimulation, although they have focused on crossmodal and bimodal aspects of auditory and visual stimulation when they report: "Simultaneous stimulation (auditory and visual) activates each cortex more strongly than the results of single stimulation and 2) After giving both auditory and visual stimuli as preliminary stimulation to each subject, only one type of stimulus was given to each subject. From this single stimulus (stimulation), both cortices (visual and auditory) were activated" (Yamamoto et al., 2004, p. 1872). .... "The [our] findings indicate that auditory and visual cortices interact with one another to a larger degree than typically assumed" (Zangenehpour & Zatorre, 2010, p. 591).

Similarly, Grahn & Rowe, (2009, p. 1231) observed that: "increases in brain activity were observed in the bilateral putamen for visual sequences preceded by auditory sequences when compared to visual sequences without prior auditory exposure" suggesting an order-dependent specificity in the effects of stimulation on neural activation.

Major increases in interest and involvement in music applications (among educators and students alike) could occur if there was sufficiently reliable evidence indicating that a combination of music and rEDLSS could improve brain functioning and learning. This would be particularly true if the improvements were in areas related to classroom learning. Although slightly lower than the IQ test score gains achieved via rEDLSS (Russell, 1996), Schellenberg (2004, 2006) has reported that 36 weeks of once weekly music lessons significantly enhanced IQ test performance in a large sample of 144 children.

Given that both rEDLSS and music appear to increase IQ test score performance, important questions for researchers in music and education could be: Would rEDLSS sessions before or during musical training increase the cognitive gains during musical training? Is there an optimum combination of rEDLSS and music for each individual that could induce the maximum amount of change in the minimum amount of time? Would increased cognitive gains interact with musical training to decrease the number of sessions required to become musically proficient? Would combining rEDLSS and music enhance cognitive performance in non-musical areas?

What is the Need for Combining rEDLSS and Music?

Alternatives to medication are always valuable, but there is a special need for alternatives when treating ADHD, given its high prevalence in young patients and the reported deleterious effects of long-term use of stimulants (the primary treatment prescribed for ADHD) in people below the age of 12. This section presents this argument in detail, starting with the nature of learning disabilities, how these disabilities are commonly treated, and the EEG correlates of ADHD. Once these characteristics have been outlined, Carter and Russell's work is presented on the use of rEDLSS to treat ADHD and other learning disabilities.

The following section details the neurological mechanisms that allow for the treatment of ADHD with this type of stimulation. Throughout the coming sections, please keep in mind that the effectiveness of rEDLSS might be increased significantly if used with music (user-selected, when possible) or when combined with music practice.

Diversity in Learning Disabilities—Attention Deficit Hyperactivity Disorder

A recent large-scale analysis by Altarac and Saroha (2007, p. S77) of data from the National Survey of Children's Health reported that the lifetime prevalence of learning disabilities (LD) in U.S. children is 9.7%. They stated that: "Although prevalence of learning disability is lower among average developing children (5.4%) it still affected 2.7 million children compared with 3.3 million (27.8%) with special health care needs. In a report from the Centers for Disease Control and Prevention (CDC, 2005, p. 842) the analysis indicated that, in 2003, approximately 4.4 million children aged 4–17 years were reported to have a history of ADHD diagnosis; of these 2.5 million children (56%) were reported to be taking medication for the disorder. Also, children in racial/ethnic minority groups and uninsured children were less likely than others to be taking medication for ADHD."

A related report (Visser, Lesesne, & Perou, 2007, p. S99) using survey data from 79,264 youths aged 4–17 states: "Nationally, 7.8% of youth aged 4–17 had a reported attention deficit disorder diagnosis and 4.3% had both a disorder diagnosis and were currently taking medication for the disorder." Additionally, the DSM-IV (4th edition) and others report that ADHD is more predominant in males (4:1) than in females (9:1). The ADHD child on average scores 7 to 15 points below their counterparts on standardized intelligence tests (Barkley, 1990). Many of the children display associated features of ADHD that include low self-esteem, depressed moods, negative perception of life, and a greater exaggeration or lability of mood (Barkley, 1990; Biederman et al., 1992; Biederman et al., 1993).

As the child matures, they are more prone to antisocial behavior (Barkley, DuPaul, & McMury, 1990; Lerner, Lowenthal, & Lerner, 1995; Waldron, 1995). Barkley et al. (1990) reported that ADHD children are three times more likely to have oppositional defiant behavior and four times more likely to exhibit conduct disorder behavior when compared to their non-ADHD peer group. In addition, the poor attention span or inattention symptoms often do not decline over time. Claude and Firestone (1995) completed a 12-year follow-up study of ADHD children/adolescents, and they concluded that individuals who have ADHD symptoms in childhood and adolescence have a greater propensity to have adult psychiatric disorders. Eighty percent of all ADHD children and adolescents will enter into adulthood with deficits in attention span, hyperactivity, and/or problems with impulsivity (Goldstein, 1997).

Although some children and adolescents show a marked decrease in problematic behavior with increasing age, most enter adulthood with inattentiveness and disorganization as the residual symptoms (Biederman et al., 1993; Lerner et al., 1995). The combination of life experiences coupled with residual problematic behavior increases the likelihood of life problems that society and the adult with ADHD will face (Barkley, 1990; Lerner et al., 1995; Goldstein, 1997).

The high concurrent rate of depression, antisocial behavior, substance abuse, and anxiety in the adult ADHD population is unparalleled in any other psychiatric disorder (Lerner et al., 1995; Goldstein, 1997). Additionally, the U.S. government recognizes ADHD as a lifelong problem through the Americans with Disabilities Act, in that payment is allowed to individuals with ADHD as a disability (Goldstein, 1997). One can easily see that problems finishing high school, poor social skills, lower self-esteem, and a greater need for mental health services for ADHD individuals and their families could be the beginning of lifelong problems (Lerner et al., 1995; Goldstein, 1997).

Behavioral Treatment and Stimulant Medication

The use of behavioral modification and/or a pharmacological intervention has been the standard treatment for the individual with ADHD. However, these forms of treatment have not proven to be overly effective (Barkley et al., 1990; Lerner et al., 1995; Waldron, 1995). Many problems exist, including:

1. Poor parenting training—implementing the behavioral treatments effectively can be difficult to teach;
2. Reluctance to place an individual on medication;
3. Side effects due to the medications;
4. Poor compliance with medications;
5. Inability to afford a pharmacological intervention;
6. The stigma placed on the individual who takes medication;
7. The poor effectiveness of both behavioral and stimulant medications for some individuals; and
8. Poor compliance with behavioral modification programs.

The most common pharmacological interventions include Methylphenidate (Ritalin©), D-amphetamine (Dexedrine©), Pemoline (Cylert©), Adderall©, Concerta©, Imipramine (Tofranil©), and Atomoxetine (Strattera©).

As the understanding of ADHD has improved over the years due to increased technology and as the diagnosing of ADHD has become more sophisticated, new forms of treatment are now emerging. Furthermore, understanding of the neurological aspects of ADHD has improved, enabling new treatment protocols. The newer forms of treatment have focused on the possibility of changing the neurological aspects of the individual with ADHD and addressing the underlying causes of their troubles, rather than just treating the symptoms. Therefore, in facing the question of possible effectiveness of different treatment protocols for the ADHD population, many researchers and clinicians have turned to the evaluation and use of newer and less invasive forms of treatment. These new forms of treatment are just now being commercialized.

Justification for Alternative Treatments

Pharmacological intervention does not come without the possibility of negative side effects. Most of the methylphenidate or dextroamphetamine-based medications for ADHD have a risk of significant side effects related to central nervous system (CNS) over-stimulation including, but not limited to, a potential for abuse of the medications. An extensive review of the medical/ scientific literature on the clinical and cost effectiveness of methylphenidate, dexamfetamine, and atomoxetine in the treatment of children and adolescents less than 18 years of age was conducted by King and colleagues in 2006 at the Center for Reviews and Dissemination, University of York, UK. They concluded that:

> "Drug therapy seems to be superior to no drug therapy; no significant differences between the various drugs in terms of efficacy or side effects were found, mainly owing to lack of evidence, and the additional benefits from behavioral therapy (in combination with drug therapy) are uncertain."

The Physicians' Desk Reference (PDR; 2007) clearly indicates that caution should be used when administering these types of drugs to individuals who have a history of drug or alcohol use and/or abuse (PDR, 2007). The prolonged use of the drugs can lead the ADHD individual to the point of abusing the drug by increasing the dosage without the physician's consent. Additional side effect can include palpitations, headaches, dyskinesia, drowsiness, blood pressure and pulse changes, tachycardia, angina, abdominal pain, weight loss, and insomnia. Individuals who use this form of pharmacological intervention for prolonged periods can also develop, in rare cases, Tourettes syndrome (PDR, 2007). The possibility of an overdose is a major concern since it can result in over-stimulation of the CNS. Overdose symptoms may include vomiting, agitation, tremors, muscle twitching, convulsions, coma, arrhythmias, and hypertension (PDR, 2007).

Another issue is that not all individuals respond to the standard behavioral treatment, and not all individuals respond to the pharmacological component of the treatment (Swanson, Kinsbourne, Roberts, & Zucker, 1978; Barkley, 1990). In addition, many individuals and their families cannot tolerate the side effects of medications (Barkley, 1990; Lerner et al., 1995; Goldstein, 1997). Furthermore, because most of the medications are Class II controlled-substance drugs, many of the parents of ADHD children and/or adolescents do not want their children on stimulant medication because of the fear of side effects or addiction to the medications. Further consideration must be given to the population of children that cannot receive treatment due to various factors such as lack of insurance, insufficient funds, and reluctance to use a pharmacological intervention.

The vast majority of past and current research has focused on symptom reduction techniques for the ADHD population, whereas the concept of changing the fundamental etiological factors or curing ADHD has not generated a great deal of research (Swanson et al., 1978; Barkley, 1990). What is remarkable is the degree of similarity between recent reviews of the efficacy of current treatments for ADHD (Swanson et al., 2007; Jensen et al., 2007; Wolraich et. al., 2005) and the findings reported in the early and middle '90's by some of the same reviewers. Various stimulant medications still offer symptomatic relief to many children with ADHD (and incur parental gratitude) and still have a number of undesirable side effects that create feelings of uncertainty and dismay in many of those same parents. Whereas many parents and people involved in treating the children are seeking alternatives, many of them may feel forced to accept the risks inherent in medications in order to get the symptomatic relief.

As the health field continues to change with the emergence of managed care and the subsequent focus on increasing the cost-effectiveness of services, it becomes imperative to search for other less intensive, more effective, and more economical ways to treat ADHD or cure it. The results of the use of programmed frequencies of audiovisual stimulation (AVS) in Micheletti's (1999) study suggests that AVS (and inferentially its successor rEDLSS) has a strong potential for being a viable treatment for ADHD individuals, providing a non-pharmacological, more economical treatment that could possibly be as effective as medication.

The individual with ADHD might eventually be able to use the treatment devices in school, at home, or in a work environment. Professional supervision is not necessary to use the AVS devices; because they are preprogrammed, they generally require less than one-half hour of training to be used properly. The rEDLSS devices do currently require adult supervision in their present research models, although there are now working versions of models suitable for home use at such time as FDA approval may be granted to make such a device commercially available. Versions of the rEDLSS are planned that will be very simple to use, safe, small, and inexpensive enough to be widely available. Whereas other rEDLSS units are available, the efficacy of their use is not known.[1]

Electroencephalographic (EEG) Differences in ADHD

At the University of Tennessee (Knoxville), Lubar's research is congruent with similar findings, including Barkley's, that an ADHD individual's EEG characteristically displays greater amounts of increased slow brainwave (theta, 4–8Hz) frequencies in their frontal and prefrontal areas when compared to non-ADHD individuals (Knights & Bakker, 1976; Lubar, 1991; Barkley, 1993; Rosenfeld, Cha, Blair, & Gotlib, 1995; Linden, Habib, & Radojevic, 1996; Sterman, 1996). Lubar and his colleagues (1985) concluded that the most important factor in the assessment of ADHD is the theta (4–8Hz) to beta (14–32Hz) ratios in the individual EEG pattern, commonly referred to as the EEG signature. Individuals who displayed ADHD characteristics had theta to beta ratios higher than those who did not display ADHD behavior. Much of this information and research was gathered by the use of quantitative EEGs (QEEG), which measures and analyzes activity from multiple leads attached to the surface of the individual's scalp (Lubar et al., 1985).

A study using single-photon emission computed tomography (SPECT) imaging found that prefrontal cortical deactivation was evident in 65% of all children and adolescents who were diagnosed with ADHD (Amen & Carmichael, 1997). The study included 54 children and adolescents who had the diagnosis of ADHD, and it measured cerebral blood flow to specific regions of the brain. Amen and Carmichael reported that the deactivation (decreased functioning) of the frontal lobe began when the individual was asked to perform a mental task. They hypothesized that this is one of the causes for the child's hyperactivity—because the child is seeking external stimulation. This deactivation hypothesis parallels Lubar's findings that when he asked a child or adolescent with ADHD to perform a mental task, his or her EEG signature would slow down (4–8Hz, theta) instead of increasing in frequency (14–32Hz, beta; Lubar et al., 1985). *Amen and his colleagues concluded that SPECT scan, PET (Positron Emission Tomography), and quantitative EEG all had clinical applications in the diagnostic phase of intervention when dealing with the ADHD population.*

As technology has improved, the basic understanding of the neurological aspect of ADHD and the treatment of the disorder has also evolved. Whereas the standard treatment (behavioral modification and medication) works well for some individuals with ADHD, many do not get properly diagnosed, fail to obtain medical help, and/or do not have the financial means to obtain the medication needed. *With the understanding that an individual who has ADHD does not have brainwaves that are behaving in the same manner as those of an individual with normal attention characteristics, the possibility of regulating brainwave patterns presents itself as a form of treatment.* This idea is not necessarily a new one. Standard stimulant medication has the effect of changing underlying EEG patterns on a temporary basis (Seifert, Scheuerpflug, Zillessen, Fallgatter, & Warnke, 2003; Rowe, Robinson, & Gordon, 2005; Sun, Wang, He, & Chen, 2007). Long-term EEG changes, however, are not the effect or intended result of stimulant treatment.

Treatment of the underlying cause(s) of the attention deficit disorders, such as developmental delays, by inducing long-lasting and positive changes in the neurological, cognitive, and behavioral functioning of children with LD/ADD/ADHD (Russell, 1996) is a primary, although, clearly a long-term goal of our working group.

How Has rEDLSS Been Studied?

Harold Russell and John Carter performed a series of experiments between 1993 and 1996 to investigate the use of rEDLSS for the short and long-term treatment of ADHD. Across five studies employing a total of 120 subjects, they consistently found that light and sound stimulation was effective in increasing IQ test scores and improving behavior in children with LD/ADD/ADHD problems. The subjects made the most cognitive improvements in their areas of lowest functioning, as measured by cognitive test scores. Given the research indicating slowed frontal EEG activity in ADHD children (Lubar, 1985, 1991, 1998), Carter and Russell (1993) speculated that the rEDLSS could be used to stimulate the brain to alternately increase and decrease EEG activity across a range of EEG frequencies.

They hypothesized that the repetitive sensory stimulation of neuronal activity, provided by rEDLSS, could result in the brain developing structural and functional changes that would enable it to shift back and forth between slower or faster processing as needed. In effect, the rEDLSS training could normalize brain functioning. Sessions could utilize the individual's dominant EEG frequency to repetitively and alternately push or pull the EEG frequency to different levels. Clinical goals can be targeted with specialized software that can rapidly calculate a percentage of the dominant frequency, and add to or subtract that amount from the dominant frequency to control the frequency of stimulation.

Initial Pilot Studies on rEDLSS

In 1993, Carter and Russell conducted a light and sound stimulation pilot study with 14 learning disabled boys from a local private school. Their mean age was 11.1 years and all showed a significant discrepancy between a verbal IQ of 116 and a non-verbal IQ of 106. None had previously been diagnosed with ADD but some or all may have qualified. Boys having a history of seizures were excluded from the study. All boys were administered the following dependent measures 1 week prior to beginning the LSS treatment and 1 week immediately following cessation of treatment: Ravens Progressive Matrices Test (RPMT), Peabody Picture Vocabulary Test-Revised (PPVT-R), Wide Range Achievement Test-Revised (WRAT-R), and the Attention Deficit Disorder Evaluation Scale-School (ADDES-S). The first group of boys received LSS treatment for 20 minutes per day, 5 days per week for 8 weeks, for a total of 40 sessions. The LSS units generated a binaural tone (see Chapter 7) synchronized with a photic stimulus from red light-emitting diodes (LED).

The frequency pattern was 10Hz for 2 minutes, 0Hz for 1 minute, 18Hz for 2 minutes, 0Hz for 1 minute and repeating until the end of 20 minutes. The frequency patterns of the binaural tones were identical to the frequencies of the LED stimulation. The sessions were designed to influence the production of beta waves in the frontal lobes of the subjects. The results indicate significant changes on four of the following variables: Ravens IQ ($p < .05$), memory ($p < .01$), reading ($p < .01$), and spelling ($p < .01$). Prior to treatment, this group had Performance IQ scores lower than their verbal scores.

Carter and Russell studied a second group of 12 learning-disabled boys at a public school. These boys received LSS training for 20 minutes per day, 5 days per week for a total of 40 training sessions. Results indicated that significant changes in two out of the six test variables were made in the Verbal area, the area of weakest functioning (WISC-R Verbal IQ $p < .05$; WRAT-R Spelling $p < .05$). A third study involved 7 experimental and 7 control subjects at another public school. This group received LSS training for 20 minutes per day, 5 days per week for 8 weeks (40 LSS sessions). The experimental group demonstrated significant improvement on three of the six variables (PPVT-R p < .05, Arithmetic p < .01, Memory p < .01). No change was seen in the control group. Once again, this study showed the pattern of improvement in the test areas with the lowest initial scores.

Based on these pilot findings, the U.S. Department of Education (USDOE/ SBIR) provided a grant (RA94130002) for a 3-year study using repetitive EEG driven light and sound stimulation (rEDLSS) as the primary intervention technique. Phase I (Russell & Carter, 1994) involved two schools, one elementary and one middle school. An equal number of boys were drawn from each school, 40 in all, as follows: 20 experimental, 10 placebo control, and 10 controls. The LD/ADD/ADHD boys were referred individually and were receiving special education services as learning disabled students. Placement into one of the three groups was random after informed consent was obtained from the parents. Boys with a personal or family history of seizure disorders were excluded. Since this was a unique treatment methodology, we believed that the study results would be clearest with a highly homogenous sample of boys only. There are well-identified gender differences with LD/ADD/ADHD, even in cross-cultural studies, including a far greater prevalence of LD/ADD/ADHD in boys than girls (Klassen, Miller, & Fine, 2004; Skounti, Philalithis, Mpitzaraki, Vamvoukas, & Galanakis, 2006; Bauermeister et al., 2007).

All boys were administered the same dependent measures used in the studies previously described. The children in the Experimental Group received the rEDLSS treatment in groups of five. Treatment time was for 22 minutes daily for 8 weeks, totaling 40 sessions. The boys were given a choice of hand held toys to play with during the sessions. The Placebo Control Group received an equal amount of time and attention in terms of educational games. The No Treatment Group was only identified and administered the pre- and post-test measures. Graduate psychology students, blind to experimental conditions and subject placement, administered all testing.

Children in the Experimental Group showed significantly greater gains in their Verbal IQ scores (approximately 10 points in 8 weeks; p < .01) than did either the Attention Placebo or the No Treatment Group. In addition, behavioral changes (decreases in inattention; p < .05) and impulsivity (p < .05) were significantly greater in the Experimental Group. The greatest improvement following the rEDLSS treatment occurred in the areas where, relatively speaking, functioning was lowest prior to training. Children with normal functioning in non-verbal areas and below-normal functioning in verbal areas (the majority of the children with LD/ADD/ADHD have this pattern) made very significant improvements in verbal functioning. The children with normal functioning in verbal areas and below normal functioning in non-verbal areas showed the most increases in non-verbal areas. This finding is in accordance with the previous reports (Carter & Russell, 1993).

SBIR Phase II Study

One goal of Phase II was to determine if the same rEDLSS treatment was equally effective with the following types of boys: neither LD nor ADD normals; LD only; LD + ADD; LD + ADHD. The same two Control, Placebo, and No Treatment groups, used in Phase I, were used for Phase II. The experimental design had 12 cells, subsumed under four major LD categories, and required 5 subjects per cell, for a total of 60 subjects. Within each of the four major categories, placement of subjects was randomized. The study design included a simple 3 X 4 ANOVA experimental design with one repeated measure during the 1st year.

A post-hoc analysis was conducted based on two age groups because research results suggested differing effects of treatment depending on age. This analysis used the oldest 25% versus the youngest 25% of the pooled sample of LD boys receiving training. Identified LD boys were placed in one of the experimental groups based upon the Home and School version of the ADDES. Once grouped, all subjects, experimental and controls, were assessed with the same dependent cognitive measures used in Phase I: the RCPM, PPVT-R, and WRAT-R. Graduate psychology students, blind to subject placement and to the experimental design, tested all the boys. All pre-testing was conducted 1 week prior to treatment. Once pre-testing was completed, the rEDLSS treatment began in the schools using school personnel trained by Russell and Carter. They employed the same training protocol as used in Phase I. The experimental group boys received 20 minutes of training, 5 days per week, for 8 weeks. Immediately upon completion of the training, all subjects were post-tested with the same measures used during pretest.

The experimental group boys received approximately 25 training sessions rather than the 40 sessions that were intended. School activities such as test days, teacher workdays, and the end of the school year precluded completion of the 40 sessions. Although the number of training sessions was only 62% of the number received in the Phase I study, significant gains were observed. The LD group showed significant improvement in both verbal and non-verbal IQ as estimated by the PPVT-R ($p < .01$) and Ravens ($p < .01$). They also showed significant improvement on the Inattention ($p < .01$) and total scores of the ADDES ($p < .01$). The ADHD group improved significantly on the Verbal ($p < .01$) and Non-Verbal ($p < .05$) IQ estimates but showed no improvement on the ADDES-S.

Training of LD/ADD Girls One of the remaining objectives of the study was to determine the effects of the rEDLSS training on school-age LD/ADD/ADHD girls. A cooperating researcher and institution (Dr. C. Chandler at the University of North Texas at Denton) was chosen to conduct this part of the research with subject selection, training, data collection, and analysis done at her institution. This study used a total of 22 girls, 10 in the experimental group and 12 controls. A summary of the findings is shown below.

Dr. Chandler employed the same training paradigm used for the boys. The girls showed significant increases on both their verbal (PPVT-R; p

Table 9.1 Summary of Data on LD/ADD Girls

Mean and SD of all dependent measures for girls

	Experimental		Control	
	Pretest	Posttest	Pretest	Posttest
PPVT-R				
Mean	90.17	95.00*	88.00	88.20
SD	15.25	14.20	6.63	5.38
RAVENS				
Mean	90.75	95.33*	98.80	96.00
SD	8.99	11.15	7.03	6.51
READING				
Mean	84.67	90.50	80.80	83.40
SD	13.81	16.35	10.11	10.84
SPELLING				
Mean	87.33	89.42	79.20	79.40
SD	13.05	13.52	6.54	11.41
ARITHMETIC				
Mean	86.42	96.58	93.00	98.00
SD	14.42	14.57	10.75	9.65

*Denotes significant .05 changes of experimental group over control group

< .05) and non-verbal IQ (Raven; $p < .05$). Achievement test score differences between the experimental and control group girls were not significant at post testing, unlike with the boys. Complete rating scales and behavioral data was unavailable due to logistical problems encountered during the study, though parents and teachers both reported a notable improvement in the girls' general sociability: shyness was reduced, willingness to participate in group activities was increased, and group situations seemed to evoke less anxiety in general, post-treatment.

Discussion of Results

A major objective of Phase II was to determine if the positive results of the rEDLSS treatment were maintained on long-term follow-up. *These results (see summary in Figure 9.2) suggest that stimulation-induced neural activation produced by the repeated use of the rEDLSS does in fact bring about long-term changes in brain functioning and behavior, rather than brief symptomatic improvement.*

Table 9.2   Summary of Posttest/Follow-up Phase II Findings

	LD ONLY	LD/ADD	LD/ADD/H
PPVT			
Posttest	.01	NS	.01
Follow-up	.01	NS	.01
RAVENS			
Posttest	.01	.01	.05
Follow-up	.01	NS	NS
READING			
Posttest	NS	NS	NS
Follow-up	.01	NS	.05
SPELLING			
Posttest	NS	NS	NS
Follow-up	.01	NS	NS
ARITHMETIC			
Posttest	NS	NS	NS
Follow-up	NS	NS	NS
INATTENTION			
Posttest	NS	.01	NS
Follow-up	NS	.01	.05
IMPULSE			
Posttest	NS	NS	NS
Follow-up	NS	NS	NS
HYPERACTIVE			
Posttest	NS	NS	NS
Follow-up	NS	NS	.05
ADDES TOTAL			
Posttest	.01	NS	NS
Follow-up	NS	.05	.01

The findings of this series of studies appear to support the concept that LD/ADD/ADHD are neurophysiologically-based disorders. The findings suggest that repeated use of this procedure (stimulation-induced neural activation), results in significant improvements on tests of cognitive functioning (IQ). *It should be noted that the LD and ADHD groups that showed significant changes at post testing on the PPVT-R maintained the changes at the same level of confidence (p < .01) at 16 months follow-up (Figure 9.2).* Additionally, the behavioral evidence available indicates improvements in attention and activity levels. Both cognitive and behavioral measures maintained this improvement at 16 months follow-up.

Although the LD/ADHD group did not show improvements at post-test on the scales of inattention and hyperactivity, they did show significant improvements on those scales at 16 months follow-up ($p < .05$, $p < .05$). The ADD group showed significant improvement on the scale of inattention at post-test ($p < .01$) and this was maintained at follow-up. This data indicates that children exposed to these stimuli make the greatest gains in their areas of lowest functioning and *also provides a strong indication that some gains continue after the treatment ends.*

Conclusions Regarding the USDOE Studies

The primary objectives of the USDOE/SBIR research were met: The first objective was to determine if the rEDLSS was an effective method of treating LD/ADD/ADHD children and adolescents. The results were consistent across the several studies within this research—significant increases were seen in both verbal and nonverbal cognitive measures, and behavior was significantly better, as rated by parents and teachers.

A second major objective was to determine if the increases found at post-testing were maintained on long-term follow-up or merely represented symptomatic gains attributable to high-technology placebo effects. The evidence appears to have been quite clear—the effects were maintained on a 16-month follow-up and there was evidence that some gains continued after treatment had ended.

The improvements in functioning found by Russell and Carter (1996) were consistent with those reported by Lubar (1995), Tansey (1993), Linden, Habib, & Radojevic (1996), and Russell (1997) using neurofeedback training. Unfortunately, neurofeedback requires expensive equipment, highly experienced technicians, and is usually administered on a one-to-one basis. rEDLSS appears to produce similar gains at a much lower cost.

The results of this series of studies suggest that rEDLSS may be a viable new treatment for attention deficit disorders in children and adolescents. So far, it appears to be an effective method of treatment (pending further confirmatory research) that is safe, low cost, and non-drug based. The possibility exists that the rEDLSS-induced increases in brain activity might interact synergistically and favorably with pharmaceutically (stimulant)-induced increases in brain activity, allowing for a reduction in medication. At present, this can only be a speculation.

There have not been any reports of negative or undesirable side effects of rEDLSS training. Many of the children have reported enjoying the training sessions. It should be noted, again, that children with a history of seizure activity or significant head injury have been excluded from the studies. The overall results form a complex pattern related to the classification of the children, that is, as LD only, LD and ADD, or LD and ADHD. The findings suggest that there may be important similarities among the children in each classification that influence the response of each group to treatment.

Accurate diagnoses are likely to be very important in establishing reasons for differential responses to treatment.

Finally, Micheletti completed a follow-up study on Russell and Carter's work for his Ph.D. dissertation at the University of Houston in 1999. He compared AVS to the effects of Ritalin in ADHD children. This study compared 99 ADHD children in four separate groups: LSS Group, LSS/Stimulant Medication Group, Stimulant Medication Group, and Self-selected Comparison Group. All groups were tested off-medication to evaluate differences at baseline. Cognitive functioning levels were evaluated by tests on the WRAT-R, PPVT-R, and Ravens. Behavioral changes were noted by the use of ADDES and the Intermediate Visual and Auditory Continuous Performance Test (IVACPT). The study evaluated the effectiveness of standard treatment of ADHD (with Ritalin© and Adderall) and the efficacy of the combination of medication and LSS treatment. All three treatment groups, (LSS Group, LSS/Stimulant Medication Group, Stimulant Medication Group), achieved significantly greater improvements on cognitive and behavioral variables, ($p < .05$, $p < .01$, and $p < .001$), when compared to the Self-selected Comparison Group. The improvements in the three treatment groups were statistically equivalent to each other, indicating equivalency of the three treatments for short-term relief of symptoms.

Teplan and colleagues (Teplan, Krakovska, & Stoic, 2006, 2011, p. 17; Teplan, Susmakova, Palus, & Vejmelka, 2009) reporting on the direct effects of long term audio-visual stimulation on EEG patterns, found indications of "increased right and left hemispheric synchronization when examined by coherence".

PART II. THE NEUROSCIENCE OF rEDLSS

How Does rEDLSS and Music Alter Brain Functioning?

Some recent research by scientists funded, in part, by the National Institute of Health (NIH), supports the following as a generalized explanation of the mechanism of action for photic and other stimulation, including auditory stimulation.

Sensory stimulation changes the brain in predictable ways (Kilgard, Pandya, Engineer,& Moucha, 2002). These changes include blood flow, metabolism, chemistry, structure, and patterns of electrical activity (Gaser & Schlaug, 1993; Lazarev, 2001). Because the neural networks within the brain resonate at specific frequencies, sensory stimulation at or near those frequencies will increase the level of activation of those networks (Narici et al., 1987; Boelen, Boelen, & Marshak, 1998; Lazarev et al., 2001). Some neuropathologies develop when certain structures in the brain are under-activated: They become locked into a state which prevents them from functioning normally, like a computer with a fast processor being throttled down by a slow system bus. These states are commonly associated with reduced blood flow and metabolism, abnormal levels of neurotransmitters, and a slowing of brainwave (EEG) frequencies (Brauchli, 1995, and Fujioka, 2010).

Inferring from the cognitive and behavioral changes observed in the USDOE studies, it is suggested that treatment with rEDLSS technology may be shifting EEG frequencies towards a more normal state. Studies from EEG scientific literature (reviewed below) have shown that key measures such as attention, memory, motor control, and cognitive performance can improve dramatically when aberrant brainwave activity "normalizes".

The following sections provide a detailed technical discussion of the evidence for this mechanism of action. Related material that was briefly touched upon in earlier sections is now examined in detail.

Intermittent Photic Stimulation, Bimodal Stimulation, and Stimulation-Induced Plasticity

The brain is capable of changing, functionally and structurally, throughout life in response to stimuli in a process known as plasticity (Johansson, 2000; Johansson, 2010; Kempermann, Van Praag, & Gage, 2000; Kilgard et al., 2001). Animal studies have shown that repetitive stimulation can cause physical changes in synaptic connections in a neural network, "thereby changing the probability of successful transmission along different pathways leading to the recorded neuron" (Bi & Poo, 1999, p. 792).

As one review of the subject stated:

"Considerable evidence supports the idea that the adult human brain maintains the ability to reorganize throughout life. This ability may underlie, at least partly, the capacity to learn and to recover from injury. The term 'plasticity,' defined as 'any enduring change in cortical properties either morphological or functional,' refers to this phenomenon. This change in cortical properties can be expressed at two interacting functional levels of the nervous system: at the level of sensory or motor cortical representation of body parts (representational or map plasticity) and at the neuronal level (neuronal or synaptic plasticity)." (Boroojerdi, Ziemann, Chen, Butefisch, & Cohen, 2001, p. 602)

A complex system of brain chemicals and hormones are involved. Neurotrophins (NT) are a family of related neurotrophic chemicals that are involved in neuronal growth such as axon path finding (Song & Poo, 1999), and synaptic plasticity (Thoenen, 1995; Angelastro et al., 2000). Increases or decreases in the levels of NTs in the brain are regulated by increases or decreases in the levels of brain or neuronal activity (Ernfors, Bengzon, Kokaia, Persson, & Lindevall, 1991; Gall & Isackson, 1989; Zafra, Hengerer, Beibrock, Thoenen, & Lindholm, 1990). NTs greatly facilitate the flow of signals across the synapses (Lohof, Ip, & Poo, 1993; Lessmann, Gottmann, & Heumann, 1994; Kang & Schuman, 1995).

Repetitive neuronal activity is thought to influence both the output of NTs and their actions (Schinder & Poo, 2000). NTs are thought to play a strong role in the modification of both the rate of synaptic transmission and the synaptic structure itself. NTs are also thought to induce long-lasting modifications (Schinder & Poo, 2000). In a review, Schinder and Poo (2000, p. 640) state that:

> "an increase or decrease of neuronal activity can enhance or reduce NT expression. Consistent with these observations, light-induced physiological activity enhanced the expression of BDNF [brain-derived neurotrophic factor] and mRNA [messenger RNA] in the visual cortex (Schinder and Poo, 2000). . . . In summary, the evidence so far strongly supports the notion that expression of BDNF and NGF [nerve growth factor] is up-regulated by electrical activity."

Other studies have indicated that additional brain hormones may modulate plasticity in the brain as a result of stimulation (Ross & Soltesz, 2001; Ziemann, Muelbacher, Hallett, & Cohen, 2001).

The electrical activity in the brain operates in a series of interconnected neural networks, which are constantly changing in response to input from other parts of the central nervous system and the peripheral nervous system. Groups of neurons operate as oscillators, which generate rhythmic electrical impulses in several frequency ranges. These oscillators are usually active in a randomized way; however by application of sensory stimulation these generators are coupled and act together in a coordinated (coherent) manner. This synchronization and enhancement of brainwave activity gives rise to "evoked" or "induced" oscillations (evoked potential; Basar, 1998, p. 211).

The result of the stimulation is described in the following:

> "if a brain structure has spontaneous rhythmic activity in a given frequency band, then this structure is tuned to the same frequency and produces internal evoked potentials to internal afferent [incoming] impulses originating in the CNS, or responds in the form of evoked potentials to external sensory stimuli with patterns similar to those of internal evoked potentials" (Basar, 1998, p. 254). "This occurs most strongly when the frequency of the stimulus is the same as the inherent frequency of the brain structures." (Boelen et al., 1998. p. 97)

Intermittent (rhythmic) photic stimulation (IPS) is particularly powerful in regards to achieving this effect. When the frequency of the IPS stimulation is very close to the naturally occurring rhythm of the visual cortex, the resulting resonance recruits and forces an increasing number of oscillators to be synchronized, and to persist in discharging in synchrony (coherently) "well after the stimulation has ceased" (Narici et al., 1987, p. 835). Photic driving can generically be described as a process of IPS inducing rhythmic brainwave activity to lock to the stimulus at a frequency identical or harmonically related to that of the stimulus (Lazarev et al., 2001).

Lazarev (2001, p. 1574) explains:

"Photic-driving can directly influence psychophysiological processes. The presence of such a response in the premotor, motor and sensorimotor cortical areas may indicate a low resistance to interference from stimulation in an individual's motor activity. Driving at the alpha frequency can produce a relaxing effect, and pronounced physiological reactions to the IPS may be observed in heart rate, breathing, galvanic skin resistance, as well as in regional cerebral blood flow."

As noted in the introduction to this chapter: "intermittent photostimulation [IPS] represents the strongest kind of stimulation among the possible sensory stimulations" (Rau, Raschka, & Koch, 2001, p. 30). This is one reason, in the view of the authors, that adding IPS to existing auditory stimulation protocols may represent a potentially dynamic, and very effective form of drug-free brain/cognitive stimulation. In addition, the brain activity levels generated by simultaneous auditory and visual stimulation are markedly greater than the sum of the effects of both auditory and visual stimulation when they are administered sequentially (Schurmann & Basar, 2000; Sakowitz, Quiroga, Schurmann, & Basar, 2001; Zangenehpour & Zatorre, 2010).

Animal research suggests a possible explanation for this effect (Wallace & Stein, 2000; Zangenehpour & Chaudhuri, 2001). There is a large group of unimodal neurons that respond only to one form of stimulation, either auditory or visual; there is a much smaller group of multimodal neurons with varying degrees of visual and auditory convergence. In these animal studies, auditory processing was largely carried out by small, bimodal groups of neurons, whereas visual processing was coordinated by both a large unimodal and a small bimodal pool of neurons. In effect, the activation of the bimodal neurons by the bimodal stimuli may account for the increased or enhanced functioning.

Many neurons are able to integrate combinations of visual, auditory, and somatosensory stimuli, markedly affecting the vigor of their responses to external stimuli (Wallace & Stein, 2001). If the cross-modal stimuli are within the multisensory neurons' receptive fields, they produce the same proportionate changes (i.e., multisensory response enhancement) when they are widely disparate as they do when they overlap on another in space (Kandunce, Vaughan, Wallace, & Stein, 2001). Multisensory neurons are thought not to simply appear at a prescribed developmental stage, but rather develop only after substantial experience with cross-modal cues (Wallace & Stein, 2001). In essence, prolonged and complex multimodal stimulation is thought to result in the development and activation of multimodal neurons that add substantially to the vigor and enhancement of brain activity (Wallace & Stein, 2001).

The complexity of continuously varying stimulation appears to be highly effective in avoiding the problem of habituation, that is, the tendency of the brain to stop responding after being presented with stimuli that are unvarying in their characteristics such as level of intensity, interval between stimuli, and content of the stimuli. In addition, "Continuously varying stimulus frequencies have the obvious virtue of allowing a better match between the frequencies of stimulation and those of latent neural oscillators [individual brain structures] than is possible with fixed frequencies" (Lazarev et al., 2001, p. 1582). Continuously varying stimulation, therefore, appears to permit a longer duration of effective stimulation at the same time that it is likely to activate more latent neural oscillators across a wide range of frequencies (Fischer, Furmark, Wik, & Fredrikson, 2000). rEDLSS stimulation frequencies are locked to the brain's fluctuating wave frequencies and therefore are continuously varying.

Similarly, music has this advantage. When it is well-crafted, it maintains the listener's attention through the variation of rhythm, intensity, timbre, and pitch. Maintaining the listener/viewer's attention seems to be crucial for stimulation to have an effect. In primate research at Johns Hopkins, Wang and colleagues (2005, p. 341) report what may be a partial explanation of the occurrence of decreased brain reactivity when a subject is presented with a boring stimulus. Specifically, they suggest that when the auditory cortex is stimulated by a [preferred] sound a particular population of neurons fire maximally throughout the duration of the sound. In contrast, responses become more transient or phasic when auditory cortex neurons respond to non-preferred stimuli. Finding stimuli that can create this response, for long periods at a stretch, blurs the lines between science, performance, therapy, and art. This is one reason why, no matter what direction this line of research takes, music will always have to be crafted by artists, those sensitive to variation, texture, and time, and those capable of skillfully and dynamically manipulating these variables in order to create a great performance. In a sense, this describes a neuroscientific basis for a great performance or great art: Those stimuli that not only grab ones attention, but hold it, are the stimuli that not only dazzle their recipient, but actually change their brain. The interesting conclusion, when one takes this and the chapter in sum, is that great art is a very healthy thing for the brain.

Brainwave Activation and Cortical Resonance

The patterns of sensory stimulation (intermittent photic and auditory stimulation) emitted by the rEDLSS evoke brainwave activation at or near the frequency of stimulation (Basar, 1998, p. 129), a phenomenon known as cortical resonance. Although it is possible to elicit larger amplitude activation at or near the alpha (8–12Hz) and theta (4–8Hz) brainwave ranges, it has recently been shown that activation can occur at frequencies up to at least 600Hz (Sannita, 2000). When various regions of the brain communicate with one another, communications pathways are established between those regions, and these remain open typically for a few tens to hundreds of milliseconds. A pathway in this sense consists of a chain of neurons, which fire one after another. This is very similar to the way information propagates through the internet—often requiring a dozen or so links between your computer and the server with the website you are accessing.

These pathways are *transient resonant systems*. They are demarcated by oscillations of the neuronal field potentials; the neurons fire in a synchronous manner at the oscillation frequency in a process called bursting (Strohmenger et al., 1997). Within the brain there are many thousands of such transient pathways being established every second. Because the various ensembles of neurons have specific resonant frequencies, they can be described as an ensemble of oscillators. Stimulation at or near the resonant frequency will increase the amplitude of resonance, in the same way that a guitar placed next to a piano will resonate with certain notes played on the piano (Basar, 1998, p. 148). The degree to which neurons are resonating together can be measured and is called coherence. If there is damage or dysfunction in the cortex, it can often be localized using a multiple electrode EEG brain map to detect aberrant coherence. The rEDLSS is capable of enhancing underutilized pathways in the brain as well as stimulating the development of new ones by measuring the coherence between two (or more) sites and establishing a stimulation protocol that will optimally select those pathways. This can be accomplished by varying the stimulation frequency while measuring the evoked response and converging on the individual's ideal frequency through (for example) successive approximations.

It is believed that this approach may also be useful for the treatment of stroke (Yamauchi et al., 2002; Johansson, 2010) and some forms of dementia, by activating quiescent pathways or creating new ones around the lesion (which typically occurs naturally, but slowly, and in an incomplete manner) due to the inherent plasticity of the brain.

Regional Cerebral Blood Flow

Inadequate blood flow to parts of the brain (hypoperfusion) is a factor in many neurological conditions. These include stroke (Grohn & Kauppinen, 2001), traumatic head injury (Sukoff, 2001), Alzheimer's disease (Suo et al., 1998; Staff et al., 2000; Mazza et al., 2010), major depression (Klemm et al., 1996; Paquette, Beauregard, Beaulieu-Prevost, 2009), and ADHD in most children (Fox & Raichle, 1985; Castellanos et al., 1996; Lou, Andresen, Steinberg, McLaughlin, & Friberg, 1998; Langleben et al., 2001; Spalletta et al., 2001). Recent studies has suggested that changes in the plasticity of the microvasculature (capillaries) of the brain related to aging may result in declines in cerebral blood flow (CBF) that reduces metabolic support for neural signaling, particularly when levels of neuronal activity are high (Riddle et al., 2003; Sonntag, Eckman, Ingralom & Riddle, 2007). Whereas this may be a subtle manifestation of inadequate blood flow, it is one that may be experienced by many people when they are tired or old and under pressure to think clearly and accurately. Current and projected developments in brain imaging methods are likely to allow accurate assessment of this possibility.

Basic neurophysiologic studies over many years have demonstrated the tight coupling between neuronal activity (the rate at which neurons emit pulses) and cerebral blood flow and metabolism (Raichle, 1987). All procedures that are known to increase the action potential frequency and excitatory postsynaptic potentials (measures of electrical charges at or in the neuron) in cortical areas are also known to increase regional cerebral blood flow (rCBF) in the same areas. This is so for motor tasks as well as somatosensory, auditory and visual stimulation (Roland, 1993).

In a PET study Fox and Raichle (1984) found that in every subject, striate cortex rCBF's percentage of change varied systematically with the rate of photic stimulation. Other studies have found that the greater the stimulation to an area of the brain the greater the metabolic response (Phelps , Kuhl, & Mazziotta, 1981; Phelps et al., 1981; Mazziotta, Phelps, Carson, & Kuhl, 1982). Kwong and colleagues (1992) have shown that photic (i.e., flickering light) stimulation can cause substantial increases in blood flow in the visual cortex. Fox and Raichle (1985) have found a similar photic stimulation rCBF response in the striate cortex. Another study used two different types of MRI methods and nine types of activation stimuli, including several types of visual stimuli, to determine that in most cases, the activation-induced increase in flow and oxygenation remained elevated for the entire stimulation duration, suggesting that both flow and oxygen consumption rates remain constant during the entire time that primary cortical neurons are activated by a task or a stimulus (Bandettini et al., 1997). More, Menon and colleagues (1992) used fMRI data obtained during photic stimulation to conclude: "neural activation increases regional cerebral blood flow (rCBF) with a concomitant increase in venous blood oxygenation" (Menon et al., 1992, p. S47).

Generally speaking, the greater the cerebral blood flow to a region, the greater the rate of cellular metabolism, and the more normal the functioning (Zametkin et al., 1990). Chiron and others (1992, p. 692), citing other investigators, have stated that:

> "It has been shown that brain development is associated with regional changes in glucose cerebral metabolic rate (rCMRG) and cerebral blood flow (rCBF). In her own study of early childhood developmental rCBF changes, Chiron reports that her results confirm that, under normal

conditions blood flow and metabolism are closely related in childhood [and her results suggest that] the development of cognitive functions is related to an rCBF increase in the corresponding cortical regions. [Further] The time needed to reach relative normal adult rCBF may be considered an index of regional maturation" (1992, p. 701).

Takahashi and colleagues (1992, p. 917) reached a similar conclusion, that: "The dynamic changes of rCBF and rCMRO2 observed in children probably reflect the physiologic developmental state within anatomic areas of the brain."

Reduced rCBF has been found in the striatum of children with ADHD (Lou et al., 1998). The striatum is an area of the brain that serves as a filter and regulator of cortical information flow (Lou, Henriksen, Bruhn, Borner, & Nielsen, 1989). In a study using positron emission tomography (PET), it was found that men who had been diagnosed with ADHD as children had lower rCBF in the corpus striatum than normal men (Schweitzer et al., 2000), an area where disorders of functioning often result in inattentiveness, distractibility, and an inability to inhibit inappropriate responses (Roland, 1993). In a study also involving ADHD, Gustafsson and his colleagues researched the association between rCBF, brainwave activity (EEG), behavioral symptoms, cognition, and neurological "soft signs" in children with ADHD. They found that the lower the rCBF in the frontal cortex, the worse *the symptoms of ADHD*; that lower rCBF in the basal ganglia correlated with motor dysfunction; and that there were at least two functionally disturbed areas of the brain in ADHD (Gustafsson, Thernlund, Ryding, Rosen, & Cederblad, 2000).

As discussed earlier, one of the major drug treatments of choice in ADHD disorder has been methylphenidate (Ritalin©), which has been reported to increase rCBF in some of the specific areas of the brain associated with short-term or working memory (Mehta et al., 2000). Part of Ritalin's effect, therefore, may possibly be of increasing the ADHD child's ability to remember what has been said to him or her long enough to respond to it appropriately. Additionally, another study of rCBF responses to methylphenidate found increased rCBF after treatment in the area of the brain known as the pathophysiologic site of ADHD (fronto-striato-thalamic circuit; Kim, Lee, Cho, & Lee, 2001).

The wide availability of brain imaging techniques allow production of images showing direct neural activation (see, e.g., Darquie, Poline, Poupon, Saint-Jalmes, & LeBihan, 2001; Draganski & Bhatia, 2010, or Tomalski & Johnson, 2010). This can allow an increasingly accurate assessment of the ability of a specific kind and pattern of stimulation to increase the levels of brain cell firing and maintain the increased levels of activity over time. Such information could be both necessary and useful in determining the degree to which the stimulation of specific music can be shown to have specific kinds of effects on brain functioning (Paquette et al., 2009).

Currently, there appears to be very little neuroimaging information linking specific musical compositions to specific changes in brain blood flow. A database of this information could be a significant aid to investigators or teachers exploring the use of music as a form of brain stimulation and brain development.

Glucose Metabolism

One of the purposes of increased blood flow in the brain is to supply oxygen, glucose, and other nutrients needed to support the metabolic activity required for increased cerebral activity. Regarding brain metabolism in adults with ADHD, one study indicated as follows:

> "In summary, we noted differences in cerebral glucose metabolism between hyperactive adults and normal adult controls, specifically in regions of the brain that have been postulated to be important in the control of preparation for motor activity, motor activity itself, inhibition of inappropriate response, and attention." (Zametkin et al., 1990, p. 1366)

Other studies have noted the abnormalities in metabolism in particular regions of the brain in ADHD subjects as compared to normal subjects (Ernst et al., 1997). Sappey-Marinier and colleagues (1992) have reported that photic stimulation not only increased cerebral blood flow but also induced a number of complex chemical changes inside the neurons, including an increased efficiency in the metabolism of glucose (glycolysis). Since glucose metabolism is the primary source of the energy the brain requires to function, an increased efficiency in glucose metabolism can translate into an ongoing increased availability of brain energy.

Preliminary Conclusions

The emphasis throughout this chapter has been on the evidence that stimulation induced neuronal activation results in significant changes and increases in human brain functioning and that the nature and extent of the changes relate to the specific nature and amount of the stimulation experienced. A special interest has been in presenting and examining the evidence that the use of two forms of brain stimulation (rEDLSS and music) may result in significant increases in cognitive performance in children as measured by IQ test scores.

A mechanism of action has been proposed that appears to be common to both rEDLSS and music. The rhythmic sensory stimulation that each modality provides results in high levels of afferent stimuli flowing into the brain. rEDLSS appears to provide high levels of discrete stimuli within a short time period that are narrowly focused into visual and auditory areas. Musical experience provides highly complex varieties of afferent stimuli flowing into the brain across a broad spectrum of sensory receptors requiring real-time integration and ongoing modifications to real-time responses while the sensory stimuli are being processed.

The significance of long-term complex musical experience may be related to the increased amount of gamma band coherence (GBC) in the EEG. This refers to an increased amount of synchronous high frequency activity present when sensory inputs from diverse areas of the brain are being rapidly processed and accurately integrated into a useful single percept. Current low-cost EEG technology permits an accurate assessment/quantification of GBC at any chosen time. For example, this could quantify the effects of either rEDLSS or musical stimulation on brain electrical activity or any desired combination of the two. If costs were not a factor, then brain-imaging data, such as fMRI, could provide excellent evidence of changes subsequent to the chosen intervention.

One of the most notable aspects of rEDLSS is the short period of time required (40, 20-minute sessions spread over 8 weeks, i.e., 800 minutes) to produce approximately a 10-point increase in IQ test scores (Russell, 1993, 1996). As reported earlier in the USDOE studies, the IQ test score gains during the second 20 sessions (5.5) were 30% greater than the gains (4.2) during the first 20 sessions. It is not known whether the scores at 60 or 80 sessions would be significantly higher than those observed at 40 sessions. Both the scientific literature and the large numbers of audiovisual stimuli pulses experienced during each session and across sessions suggest that the amount of change observed in cognitive functioning after stimulation is session or experience-dependent. To the best of the knowledge of the authors, at this time there is no systematic data to indicate the upper limits of the amount of the change in IQ test scores that may be possible for most children.

Moreover, numerous brain imaging studies have presented strong evidence that changes occur in brain structure as a result of listening to, studying, practicing, and playing music. In studies comparing the brains of highly experienced musicians to those of less experienced musicians to non-musicians, the results are again clear—the brains of highly experienced musicians with thousands of hours of practice are markedly different from those of musicians with much less experience or the brains of non-musicians. An overall impression is that musical training in its present form does result in small, although significant and long lasting gains on IQ test scores over a much longer period of training than rEDLSS. However, music will almost certainly need to become more time and cost efficient in order to gain general acceptance in schools as a method of increasing children's IQ tests scores that could enable them to increase their performance on school-related tasks.

Much more research is needed to enable the translation of these concepts and research results into information and technology that can make these procedures maximally useful in the classroom on a daily basis. The evidence presented here strongly suggests that it may be possible to bring about large and long-lasting increases in children's cognitive abilities. Schmiedek et al. (2010) commented, after reviewing the findings of numerous intervention studies on the effects of extensive practice and training on cognitive abilities, that: "(a) cognitive performance can be substantially improved through strategy training and practice up to a very old age; (b) performance gains can be maintained up to several years [and that]; (c) positive transfer of training to non-practiced tasks is generally non-existent or small."

Schmiedek et al. (2010, p. 27) comment further, however, that: "If [extensive] training does not just improve task-specific skills but also broad cognitive abilities, then even small effects could lead to important benefits for individuals' everyday intellectual competence". If the sensory stimulation of rEDLSS and music increases an individuals' cognitive abilities to learn and retain information on a long lasting basis, as it appears to do, then this increase in abilities could improve the lives of many people. As a conjecture, the long-lasting 10-point increases in IQ test scores observed in the USDOE/SBIR studies and reported in this chapter almost certainly changed the children's performance in school. Recent technological advances in computer hardware and software may make it possible for children to increase their IQ test scores more than the 10 points observed in the past. The tools and expertise exist now that can provide data-based answers to tests of this possibility.

A large free relational database (approximately 12,000 adults and 8,000 children drawn from a U.S. based population) is available through Ohio State University (the National Longitudinal Survey of Youth or NLSY). By selecting an initial group from the database with characteristics comparable or similar to those in a proposed study, the data base allows reliable estimation of what the changes would be in the proposed sample by drawing a second sample of subjects from the database differing from the first only by the amount of the expected (hypothesized) changes in the variable being studied, such as an increase in intelligence. Previous calculations have indicated that a 6-point increase in IQ (from 97 to 103) would result in a 28% decrease in permanent high school dropout rates and reduces the proportion of people who never get a high school education by 43% (Herrnstein & Murray, 1994, p. 367).[2]

Data currently exists indicating that long-lasting 10-point increases in IQ test scores are possible in LD/ADD/ADHD children. If learning disabled children can make those kinds of gains in a little over 800 minutes (less than 14 hours) of training time using the rEDLSS, could normally functioning children of average or higher levels of intelligence make even larger gains?

For the authors, one of the most intriguing questions is: What would the effects be on our educational system if most children were able to score 10 points or more higher than their current levels on IQ tests? The evidence presented in this chapter strongly suggests that such an increase is possible using currently available tools. If rEDLSS and music could enable large numbers of children to become significantly more able to learn, and an increased ability to learn was coupled with improved methods of teaching, what effect would it have on our schools, our children's lives and eventually their children's lives?

Afterword

Recently, a more advanced version of the rEDLSS was built for the first author that greatly increased its abilities to collect, analyze, display, and store training data. As a necessary part of exploring the advanced capabilities of the current version of the rEDLSS with children, he began working with and testing the capabilities of the device on himself. Reliable evidence from other investigators has shown that the brains of both humans and animals respond strongly at any age to changes and/or increases in the levels of stimulation they receive from their ongoing environment (Diamond, 1988).

The first author is 84 years old (in 2011) and in good health although he does have mild difficulties with his memory and a mild slowing of his thinking. Graphic evidence of large changes across a spectrum of frequencies in his EEG before and after using rEDLSS is intriguing and encouraging (see Figures 9.1, 9.2, 9.3). Many of the large changes observed appear to be in the higher frequency ranges, especially those frequencies usually associated with active problem solving or planning.

Examples of the changes in the frequency patterns of brain wave (EEG) activity [of the first author] before and after sensory stimulation training sessions are shown in the following figures. These figures show plots of the frequency (x-axis) ranging from 2 to 30Hz (left to right), versus the amplitude (x-axis) ranging from 0 to 40 µV. The waterfall display format plots the most recently obtained EEG in the front compared to previously obtained data progressively displayed towards the back of the plot.

Figure 9.1 shows a pre-training baseline pattern of activity, that is, before the administration of any stimulation training sessions. Note that the dominant frequency is 6.7Hz. Figure 9.2 shows the frequency patterns at the end of the 11th 20-minute training session. By this point, the dominant frequency has increased to 16.6Hz. Figure 9.3 shows the activity 25 minutes after stimulation training had ceased. The dominant frequency is 20.9Hz.

These preliminary results suggest that sensory stimulation training can induce a shift to increased activity at higher frequency levels, a result often thought to be indicative of an ability to function at higher cognitive levels. Additionally, the physiological effects of the stimulation appear to continue for some time after the training has ceased. These findings are consistent with the results of the earlier USDOE/SBIR studies indicating long-term (16-month) cognitive gains as an effect of rEDLSS training.

Subjectively, he [the first author] says that he feels much more alert after several rEDLSS sessions and that long-time colleagues comment on improvements in his thinking. Objectively, the preliminary case study data that he is collecting on himself indicates that significant upward shifts are

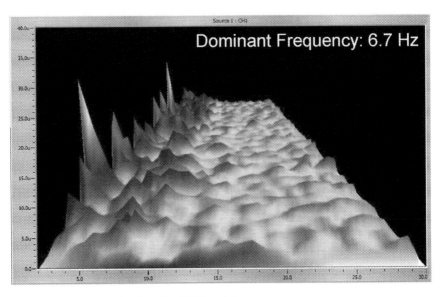

Figure 9.1 Pre-training baseline EEG activity.

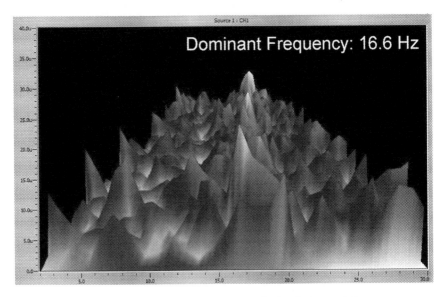

Figure 9.2 EEG activity following 20 minutes of stimulation training.

occurring in his dominant frequency activity that are observable in Figures 9.1, 9.2, and 9.3.

The single case study data thus far can only suggest that using rEDLSS to increase neural activity levels in the aging brains of older people might

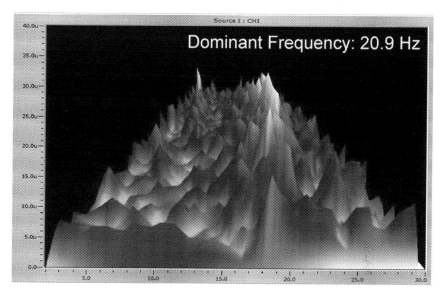

Figure 9.3   EEG activity 25 minutes after the training was discontinued.

be as helpful as it may be for the developing brains of children. Both older people and children may have similar problems with their memory, their thinking, and focusing their attention. However, it is important to remember that, although single case study data can be very interesting, systematic collection of data from larger numbers of people is needed to draw reliable evidence-based conclusions.

As a possible parallel to the changes in beta activity observed/reported above, Fujioka, Ross, Kakigi, Pantev, & Trainor (2006) have reported in MEG studies that the EEG responses of children receiving the stimulation of musical training over a 1-year period were different from those of children not receiving the musical training. A more recent report by Fujioka, Trainor, Large, & Ross (2009, p. 89) after an MEG study examining beta and gamma rhythms during passive listening to musical tones found they were "forming a periodic modulation synchronized with the stimulus [leading researchers] to propose that auditory beta and gamma oscillations have different roles in musical beat encoding and auditory-motor interaction."

Although phonological training with PC software was the specific intervention used for 6 months (10 minutes a day) with 14 dyslexic children, Penolazzi, Spironelli, Vio, & Angrilli (2010, p. 179) concluded that "those children who had the greatest reading speed enhancement showed the largest left posterior EEG beta increases." This finding suggests that increased abilities in performance may be accompanied by or related to upward shifts in brain wave frequencies. Another investigator (Gmehlin et al., 2010, p. 163) has also concluded that in school-aged children, aged 6–18:

"Normal EEG development during school age is mainly based on an absolute decrease of slow frequency activity and increases in PF [peak frequency] which may be interpreted in terms of a reorganization of the EEG towards a higher frequency oscillatory scale."

Recent data (McLaughlin et al., 2010, p. 329) indicates that children experiencing the early environmental deprivation of being reared in institutional settings "revealed significant reductions in alpha relative power and increases in theta relative power in frontal, temporal and occipital regions, suggesting a delay in cortical maturation." The accumulation of evidence presented in this chapter from current neuroplasticity research suggests that procedures that significantly increase the amount of environmental stimulation flowing into the brain results in an increase in brain maturation at any age.

Age-related deterioration in brain structure and functioning may be characterized by an absolute decrease in high(er) frequency activity and decreases in peak frequency activity which may be interpreted in terms of a reorganization of the EEG towards a lower frequency oscillatory scale. "Sensory experience plays a crucial role in developing neuronal shape and in developing synaptic contacts during brain formation . . . [and] . . . The number of synaptic contacts and the efficacy of synaptic transmission in the brain are dynamic [constantly changing] throughout development and adulthood" (Chiu & Cline, 2010, p. 2). Could it be possible that the same kind of enhancement of cognitive functioning observed in children after the prolonged, repetitive and constantly varying sensory stimulation experience of rEDLSS training and/or musical training might result in significant delays in the onset of age-related decreases in memory or other cognitive measures of brain functioning in adults?

Numerous reviews are available that summarize much of the evidence that changes in patterns of EEG activity are indicative of measurable changes in brain functioning. In turn, measurable changes in brain functioning can be useful in determining the effectiveness of procedures that result in prolonged increases in neuronal activation. Whether rEDLSS or music is used to repeatedly stimulate neuronal activity may be less important than whether the brain receives high levels of complex and interesting stimulation over a long period of time.

There is considerable interest in the concept that prolonged activity in the playing of highly interesting and engaging video games designed to require intensive involvement in rapidly changing sensory, motor and cognitive tasks may also result in increased attention spans and ability to concentrate. However, studies of this topic are in their infancy and there is considerable controversy regarding this topic.

In Summary

The existing evidence in regard to the use of rEDLSS to increase children's ability to learn is considered interesting enough by a school system in

Galveston County, Texas, that some funds have been made available and preliminary planning is underway to begin collecting data in 2011.

If the results of the studies being planned now are similar to the results of the earlier U.S. Department of Education/SBIR studies, then the results of the combined studies could be considered as evidence to justify a much larger evaluation/investigation of the benefits of the use of this technology in other schools. If funding becomes available for a larger-scale investigation of the use of rEDLSS in schools to improve children's IQ test scores, then studies are and will be planned to determine the specific combinations of rEDLSS and music that can result in the largest long-lasting IQ test score increases for most children at the lowest possible cost.

Recent research on the effects of long-term musical training (Hanna-Pladdy and Mackay, 2011) shows a high correlation between years of musical training and practice and preserved cognitive functioning in advanced age.

Lachman et al (2011) have reported (in a study involving over 3300 older subjects) that frequent cognitive activity compensates for education differences in episodic memory. In general, people with more education have been reported to have better memories than people with less education.

The evidence previously cited in this chapter indicates that the long-term and low cost use of either increased musical or rEDLSS training can improve brain functioning in children and adolescents. The results beg the following question: Is it possible that either music or rEDLSS training or some combination of procedures could enable adults to not only preserve but even improve their cognitive abilities (e.g., memory) well into advanced age, even for people as old as the first author?

A significant social and economic impact might result from a reduction in the projected costs of caring for older members of our society who experience age-related decline in brain function. Much of the current evidence that children can become "smarter" through either rEDLSS or musical training has been reviewed in this chapter. The scientific expertise and technology now exists that could provide reliable answers to questions about the effectiveness of music and rEDLSS training in improving brain function in people at different age levels. If research evidence can demonstrate that adults can gain and retain a higher level of brain function through this type of training, then it may be possible for many people (whether children or adults) to become and remain "smarter" throughout their lives. The implications of such a possibility are interesting

NOTES

1. See the Roshi© and similar devices that are capable of interfacing with a home computer. Look at Hammond, D. C. (2000). Neurofeedback treatment of depression with roshi. *Journal of Neurotherapy*, 4(2), for more information.

2. The first author has not yet calculated the dropout rate and other socio-economic effects of a 10-point or greater increase in IQ test scores using the NLSY data. There is a strong possibility that a systematic cross-correlational linking of possible or hypothesized changes in intelligence levels to possible changes in such variables as educational potentials and levels of employability could be a reference of considerable interest. It could allow some or perhaps many organizations to make more reliable estimates of the diverse socioeconomic effects of the interventions they propose. This might be particularly useful to organizations whose stated interests are in improving the physical, mental, social, and economic well being of large numbers of people.

REFERENCES

Altarac, M., & Saroha, E. (2007). Lifetime prevalence of learning disability among US children. *Pediatrics, 119*(Supplement 1), S77–83.

Amen, D. G., & Carmichael, B. D. (1997). Evaluating with brain SPECT imaging. *Biofeedback, 25,* 4.

Angelastro, J. M., Klimaschewski, L., Tang, S., Vitolo, O. V., Weissman, T. A., Donlin, L. T., . . . Greene, L. A. (2000). Identification of diverse nerve growth factor-regulated genes by serial analysis of gene expression (SAGE) profiling. *Proceedings of the National Academy of Sciences USA, 97,* 10424–10429.

Bandettini, P. A., Kwong, K. K., Davis, T. L., Tootell, R. B., Wong, E. C., Fox, P. T., . . . Rosen, B. R. (1997). Characterization of cerebral blood oxygenation and flow changes during prolonged brain activation. *Human Brain Mapping, 5,* 93–109.

Barkley, R. A. (1990). *Attention Deficit Hyperactivity Disorder: A handbook for diagnosis and treatment.* New York: The Guilford Press.

Barkley, R. A. (1993). A new theory of ADHD. *The ADHD Report, 1,* 1–4.

Barkley, R. A., Anastopoulos, A. D., Guevremont, D. C., & Fletcher, K. E. (1991). Adolescents with ADHD: Patterns of behavioral adjustment, academic functioning, and treatment utilization. *Journal of the American Academy of Child and Adolescent Psychiatry, 30,* 752–753.

Barkley, R. A., DuPaul, G. J., & McMury, M. B. (1990). Comprehensive evaluation of attention deficit disorder with and without hyperactivity as defined by research criteria. *Journal of Consulting and Clinical Psychology, 58,* 775–789.

Basar, E. (1998). *Brain function and oscillations. Volume I: Brain oscillations. Principles and approaches* (pp. 129–254). Berlin: Springer.

Bauermeister, J. J., Shrout, P. E., Chavez, L., Rubio-Stipec, M., Ramirez, R., Padilla, L., . . . Canino, G. (2007). ADHD and gender: Are risks and sequelae of ADHD the same for boys and girls? *Journal of Child PsycholPsychiatry, 48*(8), 831–839.

Bi, G., & Poo, M. (1999). Distributed synaptic modification in neural networks induced by patterned stimulation. *Nature, 401,* 792–796.

Biederman, J., Faraone, S. V., Keenan, K., Benjamin, J., Krifcher, B., Moore, C., . . . Tsuang, M. T. ((1992). Further evidence for family-genetic risk factors in attention deficit hyperactivity disorder. *Archives of General Psychiatry, 49,* 728–737.

Biederman, J., Faraone, S. V., Spencer, T., Wilens, T., Norman, D., Lapey, K. A., . . . Doyle, A. (1993). Patterns of psychiatric comorbidity, cognition, and psychosocial functioning in adults with attention deficit hyperactivity disorder. *American Journal Psychiatry, 12,* 1792–1797.

Biederman, J., & Spencer, T. (1999). Attention-deficit/hyperactivity disorder (ADHD) as a noradrenergic disorder. *Biological Psychiatry, 46*, 1234–1242.

Boelen, M. K., Boelen, M. G., & Marshak, D. W. (1998). Light-stimulated release of dopamine from the primate retina is blocked by l-2-amino-4-phosphonobutyric acid (APB). *Visual Neuroscience, 15*, 97–103.

Boroojerdi, B., Ziemann, U., Chen, R., Butefisch, C. M., & Cohen, L. G. (2001). Mechanisms underlying human motor system plasticity. *Muscle Nerve, 24*, 602–613.

Brandt, S. A., Brocke, J., Roricht, S., Ploner, C. J., Villringer, A., & Meter, B. U. (2001). In vivo assessment of human visual system connectivity with transcranial electrical stimulation during functional magnetic resonance imaging. *Neuroimage, 14*(2), 366–375.

Brauchli, P., Michel, C. M., & Zeier, H. (1995). Electrocortical, autonomic, and subjective responses to rhythmic audio-visual stimulation. *International Journal of Psychophysiology, 19*(1), 53–66.

Brockhuis, B., Slawek, J., Wieczorek, D., Ussorowska, D., Derejko, M., Romanowicz, G., . . . Dubaniewicz, M. (2006). Cerebral blood flow changes in patients with dementia with Lewy bodies (DLB). A study of 6 cases. *Nuclear Medicine Review, Central & Eastern Europe 9*(2), 114–118.

Brown, J. T., Davies, C. H., & Randall, A. D. (2007). Synaptic activation of GABA(B) receptors regulates neuronal network activity and entrainment. *European Journal of Neuroscience, 25*(10), 2982–2990.

Cappe, C., Thut, G., Romel, V., & Murray, M. M. (2010). Auditory-visual multisensory interactions in human timing, topography, directionality, and sources. *Journal of Neuroscience, 30*(38), 12572–12580.

Carter, J. L., & Russell, H. L. (1993a). *An audiovisual stimulation unit with EEG biofeedback for treatment of learning disabilities.* First Annual Report, U.S. Department of Education/SBIR, Phase II, Contract No. RA 94130002.

Carter, J. L., & Russell, H. L. (1993b). A pilot investigation of auditory and visual entrainment of brain wave activity in learning disabled boys. *Texas Researcher, 4*, 65–73.

Carter, J., & Russell, H. (1995). *An EEG driven light sound stimulation unit for enhancing cognitive abilities of learning disabled boys.* Sixth Annual Report, U.S. Department of Education/SBIR, Phase II, Contract No. RA 94130002.

Carter, J., & Russell, H. (1996). *An EEG-driven lightsound stimulation unit for enhancing cognitive abilities in learning disabled boys.* Final Report, U.S. Department of Education/SBIR, Phase II Contract No. 94130002.

Castellanos, F. X., Giedd, J. N., Marsh, W. L., Hamburger, S. D., Vautuzis, A. C., Dickstein, D. P., . . . Centers for Disease Control and Prevention (CDC). (2005). Mental health in the United States. Prevalence of diagnosis and medication treatment for attention-deficit/hyperactivity disorder–United States, 2003. *Morbidity and Mortality Weekly Report, 54*(34), 842–847.

Chiron, C., Raynaud, C., Mazire, B., Zilbovicius, M., Laflamme, L., Masure, M. C., . . . Syrota, A. (1992). Changes in regional cerebral blood flow during brain maturation in children and adolescents. *Journal of Nuclear Medicine, 33*(5), 696–703.

Chiu, S. L. Cline H. T. Insulin Receptors Signaling in the Development of Neuronal Structures and Functioning. *Neural Development.* Pub online 2010 March 15.

Claude, D., & Firestone, P. (1995). The development of ADHD boys: A 12-year follow-up. *Canadian Journal of Behavioral Science, 27*, 226–249.

Darquie, A., Poline, J. B., Poupon, C., Saint-Jalmes, H., & Le Bihan, D. (2001). Transient decrease in water diffusion observed in human occipital cortex during visual stimulation. *Proceedings of the National Academy of Sciences USA, 98*, 9391–9395.

Diamond, A. (1988). Abilities and neural mechanisms underlying AB performance. *Child Development, 59*(2), 523–527.

Diamond, M. C. (2001). Response of the brain to enrichment. *An Acad Bras Cienc, 73*(2), 211–220.

Draganski, B., & Bhatia, K. P. (2010). Brain structures in movement disorders: A neuroimaging perspective. *Current Opinions in Neurology, 23*(4), 413–419.

Duffy, F. H., Iyer, V. G., & Surwillo, W. W. (1989). *Clinical electroencephalography and topo-graphic brain mapping. Technology and practice.* Ann Arbor, MI: Edwards Brothers, Inc.

Eriksson, E. (1999). Serotonin reuptake inhibitors for the treatment of premenstrual dysphoria. *International Clinical Psychopharmacology, 14*(Supplement 2), 27–33.

Eriksson, E., Andersch, B., Ho, H. P., Landen, M., & Sundblad, C. (2001). Serotonin uptake inhibitors provide rapid relief from premenstrual dysphoria. New findings shed light on how serotonin modulates sex hormone-related behavior. *Lakartidningen, 98*(34), 3524–3530.

Ernfors, P., Bengzon, J., Kokaia, Z., Persson, H., & Lindvall, O. (1991). Increased levels of messenger RNAs for neurotrophic factors in the brain during kindling epileptogenesis. *Neuron, 7,* 165–176.

Ernst, M., Cohen, R. M., Liebenauer, L. L., Jons, P. H., & Zametkin, A. J. (1997). Cerebral glucose metabolism in adolescent girls with attention-deficit/hyperactivity disorder. *Journal of the American Academy of Child Adolescent Psychiatry, 36,* 1399–1406.

Ernst, M., Zametkin, A. J., Matochik, J. A., Pascualvaca, D., Jons, P. H., & Cohen, R. M. (1999). High midbrain [18F] DOPA accumulation in children with attention deficit hyperactivity disorder. *American Journal of Psychiatry, 156,* 1209–1215.

Ferrier, I. N. (2001). Characterizing the ideal antidepressant therapy to achieve remission. *Journal of Clinical Psychiatry, 62*(Supplement 26), 10–15.

Fjell, A. M., & Walhovd, K. B. (2010). Structural brain changes in aging: Courses, causes and cognitive consequences. *Reviews in the Neurosciences, 21*(3), 187–221.

Fischer, H., Furmark, T., Wik, G., & Fredrikson, M. (2000). Brain representation of habituation to repeated complex visual stimulation studied with PET. *NeuroReport, 11*(1), 123–126.

Fischman, A. J., Bonab, A. A., Babich, J. W., Palmer, E. P., Alpert, N. M., Elmaleh, D. R., . . . Madra, B. K. (1998). Rapid detection of Parkinson's disease by SPECT with altropane: A selective ligand for dopamine transporters. *Synapse, 29*(2), 128–141.

Forgeand, M. Winner, E., Norton, A. & Schlang, G. 2008. Practicing a Musical Instrument in Childhood is Associated with Enhanced Verbal Ability and Nonverbal Reasoning. *Plus One 3(10):* 3566

Fox, P. T., & Raichle, M. E. (1984). Stimulus rate dependence of regional cerebral blood flow in human striate cortex, demonstrated by positron emission tomography. *Journal of Neurophysiology, 51,* 1109–1120.

Fox, P. T., & Raichle, M. E. (1985). Stimulus rate determines regional blood flow in striate cortex. *Annals of Neurology, 17,* 303–305.

Fujioka, T., Ross, B., Kakigi, R., Pantev, C., & Trainor, L. J. (2006). One year of musical training affects development of auditory cortical-evoke field. *Brain, 129*(Part 10), 2593–2608.

Fujioka, T., Trainor, L. J., Large, E. W., & Ross, B. (2009). Beta and gamma rhythms in human auditory cortex during musical beat processing. *Annals of the New York Academy of Sciences, 1169,* 89–92.

Gall, C. M., & Isackson, P. J. (1989). Limbic seizures increase neuronal production of messenger RNA for nerve growth factor. *Science, 245,* 758–761.

Gaser, C., & Schlaug, G. (2003). Brain structures differ between musicians and non-musicians. *Journal of Neuroscience, 23*(27), 9240–9245.

Gmehlin, D. Thomas, C. Weisbrod, M., Walther, S., Pfuller, U., Resch, F., & Aelkers-Ax, R. 2011. Individual Analysis of EEG Background-Activity Within School Age: Impact of Age and Sex Within a Longitudinal Data Set. *International Journal of Developmental Neuroscience.* Apr. 29(2): 163-70. Epub 2010 Dec. 4.

Goldstein, S. (1997). *Managing attention and learning disorders in late adolescence and adulthood.* New York: Wiley Interscience Press.

Grahn, J. A., Henry, M. J., & McAuley, J. D. (2011). FMRI investigation of cross-modal interactions in beat perception: Audition primes vision, but not vice versa. *Neuroimage, 54*(2), 1231–1243.

Grahn, J. A., & Rowe, J. B. (2009). Feeling the beat: Premotor and striatal interactions in musicians and nonmusicians during beat perception. *Journal of Neuroscience, 29*(23), 7540–7548.

Graziano, A. B., Peterson, M., & Shaw, G. L. (1999). Enhanced learning of proportional math through music training and spatial-temporal training. *Neurological Research, 21*(2), 139–152.

Grohn, O. H., & Kauppinen, R. A. (2001). Assessment of brain tissue viability in acute ischemic stroke by BOLD MRI. *NMR Biomed, 14*(7–8), 432–440.

Groussard, M., La Joie, R., Rauchs, G., Landau, B., Chetelat, G., Viader, F., . . . Platel, H. (2010). When music and long-term memory interact: Effects of musical expertise on functional and structural plasticity in the hippocampus. *PLoS One, 5*(10), pii e13225.

Gustafsson, P., Thernlund, G., Ryding, E., Rosen, I., & Cederblad, M. (2000). Associations between cerebral blood-flow measured by single photon emission computed tomography (SPECT), electro-encephalogram (EEG), behavior symptoms, cognition and neurological soft signs in children with attention-deficit hyperactivity disorder (ADHD). *Acta Paediatr, 89*, 830–835.

Hale, T. S., Hariri, A. R., & McCracken, J. T. (2000). Attention-deficit/hyperactivity disorder: Perspectives from neuroimaging. *Mental Retardation Developmental Disability Research Reviews*, 6, 214–219.

Hallowell, E. M., & Ratey, J. J. (1994). *Driven to distraction.* New York: Pantheon Books.

Hanna-Pladdy, B., Mackay, A. 2011. The Relation Between Instrumental Musical Activity and Cognitive Aging. *Neuropsychology.* 2011. Apr 4.

Herrnstein, R. J., & Murray, C. (1994). *The Bell Curve* (pp. 120, 366). New York: Free Press.

Hodes, R. L. (1989). The biofeedback treatment of neurological and neuropsychological disorders of childhood and adolescence. In C. R. Reynolds, E. Fletcher-Janzen (Eds.), *Handbook of clinical child neuropsychology* (pp. 337–396). New York: Plenum Press.

Hoeft, F., McCandless, B. D., Black, J. M., Gantman, A., Zakerant, N., Hulme, C., . . . Gabrieli, J. D. E. (2010). Neural systems predicting long-term outcome in dyslexia. *Proceedings of the National Academy of Sciences USA.* Epub December 20, 2010.

Holtzman, T., Rajapaksa, T., Mostofi, A., & Edgley, S. A. (2006). Different responses of rat cerebellar Purkinje cells and Golgi cells evoked by widespread convergent sensory inputs. *Journal of Physiology, 574*(Part 2), 491–507. Epub May 18, 2006.

Hu, M., Retz, W., Baader, M., Pesold, B., Adler, G., Henn, F. A., . . . Thome, J. (2000). Promoter polymorphism of the 5-HT transporter and Alzheimer's Disease. *Neuroscience Letters, 294*(1), 63–65.

Hyder, F., Kida, I., Behar, K. L., Kennan, R. P., Maciejewski, P. K., & Rothman, D. L. (2001). Quantitative functional imaging of the brain: Towards mapping neuronal activity by BOLD fMRI. *NMR Biomed, 14*(7–8), 413–431.

Jensen, P. S., Arnold, L. E., Swanson, J. M., Vitiello, B., Abikoff, H. B., Greenhill, L. L., . . . Hur, K. (2007). 3-year follow-up of the NIMH MTA study. *Journal of the American Academy of Child Adolescent Psychiatry, 46*(8), 989–1002.

Johansson, B. B. (2000). Brain plasticity and stroke rehabilitation. The Willis Lecture. *Stroke, 31,* 223–230.

Johansson, B. B. (2003). Neurorehabilitation and brain plasticity. *Journal of Rehabilitation Medicine, 35*(1), 1.

Johansson, B. B. (2004). Brain plasticity in health and disease. *Keio Journal of Medicine, 53*(4), 231–246. Review.

Johansson, B. B. (2007). Regeneration and plasticity in the brain and spinal cord. *Journal of Cerebral Blood Flow & Metabolism, 27*(8), 1417–1430. Epub March 28.

Johanssson, B. B. (2010). Current trends in stroke rehabilitation: A review with focus on brain plasticity. *Acta Neurol Scand,* August 19, 2010.

Kandunce, D. C., Vaughan, J. W., Wallace, M. T., & Stein, B. E. (2001).The influence of visual and auditory receptive field organization on multisensory integration in the superior colliculus. *Experimental Brain Research, 139*(3), 303–310.

Kang, H., & Schuman, E. M. (1995). Long-lasting neurotrophin-induced enhancement of synaptic transmission in the adult hippocampus. *Science, 267,* 1658–1662.

Kaur, G., & Kulkarni, S. K. (2001). Investigations on possible serotonergic involvement in effects of OB-200G (polyherbal preparation) on food intake in female mice. *European Journal of Nutrition, 40*(3), 127–133.

Kempermann, G., Van Praag, H., & Gage, F. H. (2000). Activity-dependent regulation of neuronal plasticity and self repair. *Prog. in Brain Res, 127,* 35–48.

Kilgard, M. P., & Merzenich, M. M. (2002). Order-sensitive plasticity in adult primary auditory cortex. *Proceedings of the National Academy of Sciences USA, 99*(5), 3205–3209.

Kilgard, M. P., Pandya, P. K., Engineer, N. D., & Moucha, R. (2002). Cortical network reorganization guided by sensory input features. *Biological Cybernetics, 87*(5–6), 333–343.

Kilgard, M. P., Pandya, P. K., Vazquez, J., Gehi, A., Schreiner, C. E., & Merzenich, M. M. (2001). Sensory input directs spatial and temporal plasticity in primary auditory cortex. *Journal of Neurophysiology, 86,* 326–338.

Kim, B. N., Lee, J. S., Cho, S. C., & Lee, D. S. (2001). Methylphenidate increases regional cerebral blood flow in subjects with attention deficit/hyperactivity disorder. *Yonsei Medical Journal, 42,* 19–29.

Kim, J. K., & Zatorre, R. J. (2010). Can you hear shapes you touch? *Experimental Brain Research, 202*(4), 747–754.

King, S., Griffin, S., Hodges, Z., Weatherly, H., Asseburg, C., Richardson, G., . . . Riemsma, R. (2006). A systematic review and economic model of the effectiveness and cost-effectiveness of methylphenidate, dexamfetamine and atomoxetine for the treatment of attention deficit hyperactivity disorder in children and adolescents. *Health Technology Assessment, 10*(23), iii–iv, xiii–146.

Klassen, A. F., Miller, A., & Fine, S. (2004). Health-related quality of life in children and adolescents who have a diagnosis of attention-deficit/hyperactivity disorder. *Pediatrics, 114*(5), e541–547.

Klemm, E., Danos, P., Grunwald, F., Kasper, S., Moller, H. J., & Biersack, H. J. (1996). Temporal lobe dysfunction and correlation of regional cerebral blood flow abnormalities with psychopathology in schizophrenia and major depression—a study with single photon emission computed tomography. *Psychiatry Research, 68*(1), 1–10.

Klingberg, T. (2010). Training and plasticity of working memory. *Trends in Cognitive Science, 14*(7), 317–324.

Knights, R. M., & Bakker, D. J. (1976). *The neuropsychology of learning disorders theoretical approaches.* Baltimore, MA: University Park Press.

Kolb, B. (2003). Overview of cortical plasticity and recovery from brain injury. *Physical Medicine and Rehabilitation Clinics of North America, 14*(Supplement 1), S7–25, viii.

Komitova, M., Johansson, B. B., & Eriksson, P. S. (2006). On neural plasticity, new neurons and the post-ischemic milieu: An integrated view on experimental rehabilitation. *Experimental Neurology, 199*(1), 42–55. Epub 2006 Apr 24.

Krause, K. H. Dresel, S. H., Krause, J., Kung, H. F., & Tatsch, K. (2000). Increased striatal dopamine transporter in adult patients with attention deficit hyperactivity disorder: Effects of methylphenidate as measured by a single photon emission computed tomography. *Neuroscience Letters, 285*, 107–110.

Kwong, K. K., Belliveau, J. W., Chesler, D. A., Goldberg, I. E., Weisskoff, R. M., Poncelet, B. P., . . . Turner, R. (1992). Dynamic magnetic resonance imaging of human brain activity during primary sensory stimulation. *Proceedings of the National Academy of Sciences USA, 89*, 5675–5679.

Lam, R. W., Tam, E. W., Grewal, A., & Yatham, L. N. (2001). Effects of alpha-methyl-para-tyrosine-induced catecholamine depletion in patients with seasonal affective disorder in summer remission. *Neuropsychopharmacology, 25*(Supplement 5), 97–101.

Lane, J. D., Kasian, S. J., Owens, J. E., & Marsh, G. R. (1998). Binaural auditory beats affect vigilance performance and mood. *Physiology and Behavior, 63*(2), 249–252.

Langleben, D. D., Austin, G., Krikorian, G., Ridlehuber, H. W., Goris, M. L., & Strauss, H. W. (2001). Interhemispheric asymmetry of regional cerebral blood flow in prepubescent boys with attention deficit hyperactivity disorder. *Nuclear Medicine Communications, 22*(12), 1333–1340.

Lazarev, V. V., Simpson, D. M., Schubsky, B. M., & DeAzevedo, L. C. (2001). Photic driving in the electroencephalogram of children and adolescents: Harmonic structure and relation to the resting state. *Brazilian Journal of Medical and Biological Research, 34*(12), 1573–1584.

Lerner, J. W., Lowenthal, B., & Lerner, S. R. (1995). *Attention deficit disorders.* New York: Brooks/Cole Publishing Company.

Lessmann, V., Gottmann, K., & Heumann, R. (1994). BDNF and NT4/5 enhance gluta-matergic synaptic transmission in cultured hippocampal neurones. *NeuroReport, 6*, 21–25.

Levitin, D. J. (2005). Musical behavior in a neurogenetic developmental disorder: Evidence from Williams Syndrome. *Annals of the New York Academy of Sciences, 1060*, 325–334.

Linden, M., Habib, T., & Radojevic, V. (1996). A controlled study of the effects of EEG biofeedback on cognition and behavior of children with attention deficit disorder and learning disabilities. *Biofeedback and Self-Regulation, 21*, 35–49.

Lohof, A. M., Ip, N. Y., & Poo, M. M. (1993). Potentiation of developing neuromuscular synapses by the neurotrophins NT3 and BDNF. *Nature, 363*, 350–353.

Lou, H. C., Andresen, J., Steinberg, B., McLaughlin, T., & Friberg, L. (1998). The striatum in a putative cerebral network activated by verbal awareness in normals and in ADHD children. *European Journal of Neurology, 5*, 67–74.

Lou, H. C., Henriksen, L., Bruhn, P., Borner, H., & Nielsen, J. B. (1989). Striatal dysfunction in Attention Deficit and Hyperkinetic Disorder. *Archives of Neurology, 46*, 48–52.

Lou, H. C., Rosa, P., Pryds, O., Karrebaek, H., Lunding, J., Cumming, P., & Gjedde, A. (2004). ADHD: Increased dopamine receptor availability linked to attention deficit and low neonatal cerebral blood flow. *Dev Med Child Neurol, 46*(3), 179–183.

Lubar, J. F. (1991). Discourse on the development of EEG diagnostics and biofeedback for attention-deficit hyperactivity disorder. *Biofeedback and Self-Regulation, 16*, 201–225.

Lubar, J. F. (1998). Electroencephalographic biofeedback methodology and the management of epilepsy. *Integrative Physiological and Behavioral Science, 23*, 243–263.

Lubar, J. F., Bianchini, K. J., Calhoun, W. H., Lambert, E. W., Brody, A. H., & Shabsin, H. S. (1985). Spectral analysis of EEG differences between children with and without learning disabilities. *Journal of Learning Disabilities, 18*, 403–408.

Marshall, R. S., Ferrera, J. J., Barnes, A., Zhang, X., O'Brien, K. A., Chmayssani, M., . . . Lazar, R. M. (2007). Brain activity associated with stimulation therapy of the visual border zone in hemianopic stroke patients. *Neurorehabilitation and Neural Repair*. Epub ahead of print. August 15, 2007.

Mazza, M., Marano, G., Traversi, G., Bria, P., & Mazza, S. (2010). Primary cerebrak blood flow deficiency and Alzheimer's disease: Shadows and lights. *Journal of Alzheimer's Disease*. Epub ahead of print. November 23.

Mazziotta, J. C., Phelps, M. E., Carson, R. E., & Kuhl, D. E. (1982). Tomographic mapping of human cerebral metabolism: Auditory stimulation. *Neurology, 32*, 921–937.

McDonnell, M. N., Hillier, S. L., Miles, T. S., Thompson, P. D., & Ridding, M. C. (2007). Influence of combined afferent stimulation and task-specific training following stroke: A pilot randomized controlled trial. *Neurorehabilitation and Neural Repair, 21*(5), 435–443. Epub April 3, 2007.

McLaughlin, K. A., Fox, N. A., Zeanah, C. A. Sheridan, M. A., Marshall, P., Nelson, C. A. 2010. Delayed Maturation in Brain Electrical Activity Partially Explains the Association Between Early Environmental Deprivations and Symptoms of Attention Deficit Hyperactivity Disorders. *Biological Psychiatry*. Aug. 15: 68(4): 329–36. Epub. 2010 May 23.

Mehta, M. A., Owen, A. M., Sahakian, B. J., Mavaddat, N., Pickard, J. D., & Robbins, T. W. (2000). Methylphenidate enhances working memory by modulating discrete frontal and parietal lobe regions in the human brain. *Journal of Neuroscience, 20*, RC65.

Menon, R. S., Ogawa, S., Kim, S. G., Ellermann, J. M., Merkle, H., Tank, D. W., & Ugurbil, K. (1992). Functional brain mapping using magnetic resonance imaging. Signal changes accompanying visual stimulation. *Invest Radiol, 27*(Supplement 2), S47–53.

Meyer, J. H., Kruger, S., Wilson, A. A., Christensen, B. K., Goulding, V. S., Schaffer, A., & Kennedy, S. H. (2001). Lower dopamine transporter binding potential in striatum during depression. *Neuroport, 12*(18), 4121–4125.

Micheletti, L. (1999). *The use of light and sound stimulation for the treatment of attention deficit hyperactivity disorder in children*. Dissertation, University of Houston, Houston, Texas.

Miles, T. S., Ridding, M. C., McKay, D., & Thompson, P. D. (2005). Motor cortex excitability after thalamic infarction. *Journal of Clinical Neuroscience, 12*(4), 469–472.

Miller, G. M., De La Garza, R. D. II, Novak, M. A., & Madras, B. K. (2001). Single nucleotide polymorphisms distinguish multiple dopamine transporter alleles in primates: Implications for association with attention deficit hyperactivity disorder and other neuropsychiatric disorders. *Molecular Psychiatry, 6*, 50–58.

Mito, Y., Yoshida, K., Yabe, I., Makino, K., Hirotani, M., Tashiro, K., . . . Sasaki, H. (2005). Brain 3D-SSP SPECT analysis in dementia with Lewy bodies, Parkinson's disease with and without dementia, and Alzheimer's disease. *Clinical Neurology and Neurosurgery, 107*(5), 396–403. Epub January 19, 2005.

Mori, S. (2002). Responses to donepezil in Alzheimer's disease and Parkinson's disease. *Annals of the New York Academy of Sciences, 977*, 493–500.

Narici, L., Romani, G. L., Salustri, C., Pissella, V., Modena, I., & Papanicolaou, A. C. (1987). Neuromagnetic evidence of synchronized spontaneous activity in the brain following repetitive sensory stimulation. *International Journal of Neuroscience, 32*, 831–836.

Neumeister, A., Willeit, M., Praschak-Rieder, N., Asenbaum, S., Stastny, J., Hilger, E., . . . Kasper, S. (2001). Dopamine transporter availability in symptomatic depressed patients with seasonal affective disorder and healthy controls. *Psychological Medicine, 31*(8), 1467–1473.

Ors, M., Ryding, E., Lindgren, M., Gustafsson, P., Blennow, G., & Rosen, I. (2005). SPECT findings in children with specific language impairment. *Cortex, 41*(3), 316–326.

Pantev, C., Ross, B., Fujioka, T., Trainor, L. J., Schulte, M., & Schulz, M. (2003). Music and learning-induced cortical plasticity. *Annals of the New York Academy of Sciences, 999*, 438–450. Review.

Paquette, V., Beauregard, M., & Beaulieu-Prevost, D. (2009). Effect of a psychoneurotherapy on brain electromagnetic tomography in individuals with major depressive disorder. *Psychiatry Research, 174*(3), 231–239.

Pastor, M. A., Artieda, J., Arbizu, J., Marti-Climent, J. M., Penuelas, I., & Masdeu, J. C. (2002). Activation of human cerebral and cerebellar cortex by auditory stimulation at 40 Hz. *Journal of Neuroscience, 22*(23), 10501–10506.

Pastor, M. A., Artieda, J., Arbizu, J., Valencia, M., & Masdeu, J. C. (2003). Human cerebral activation during steady-state visual-evoked responses. *Journal of Neuroscience, 23*(37), 11621–11627.

Patz, S., & Wahle, P. (2004). Neurotrophins induce short-term and long-term changes of cortical neurotrophin expression. *European Journal of Neuroscience, 20*(3), 701–708.

Penolazzi, B., Spironelli, C., Vio, C., & Angrilli, A. (2010). Brain plasticity in developmental dyslexia after phonological treatment: a beta EEG band study. *Behavioral Brain Research, 209*(1), 179–182.

Peretz, I., & Zatorre, R. J. (2005). Brain organization for music processing. *Annual Review of Psychology, 56*, 89–114. Review.

Peretz, I., Gosselin, N., Belin, P. Zatorre, J., Plailly, J., Tillma, B. 2009. Music Lexical Networks: the Cortical Organization of Music Recognition. Annals New York Academy of Science. Jul.; 1169: 256–65.

Peterson, D. A., & Thaut, M. H. (2007). Music increases frontal EEG coherence during verbal learning. *Neuroscience Letters, 412*(3), 217–221.

Phelps, M. E., Kuhl, D. E., & Mazziota, J. C. (1981). Metabolic mapping of the brain's response to visual stimulation: Studies in humans. *Science, 211*, 1445–1448.

Phelps, M. E., Mazziotta, J. C., Kuhl, D. E., Nuwer, M., Packwood, J., Metter, J., & Engel, J. (1981). Jr. Tomographic mapping of human cerebral metabolism visual stimulation and deprivation. *Neurology, 31*, 517–529.

Physicians Desk Reference. (PDR). (2007). Montvale, NJ: Medical Data Production Company.

Pleger, B., Foerster, A. F., Widdig, W., Henschel, M., Nicolas, V., Jansen, A., . . . Tegenthoff, M. (2003). Functional magnetic resonance imaging mirrors recovery of visual perception after repetitive tachistoscopic stimulation in patients with partial cortical blindness. *Neuroscience Letters, 335*(3), 192–196.

Raichle, M. E. (1987). Circulatory and metabolic correlates of brain function in normal humans. In *Handbook of physiology–The nervous system* (Vol. 5; pp. 643–674). American Physiological Society.

Rajapakse, J. C., & Rapoport, J. L. (1996). Quantitative brain magnetic resonance imaging in attention-deficit hyperactivity disorder. *Archives of General Psychiatry, 53*, 607–616.

Rau, R., Raschka, C., & Koch, H. J. (2001). Phenomena of intermittent rhythmic photostimulation in neuronal plasticity. *Nagoya Journal of Medical Science, 64*(1–2), 19–32.

Rauscher, F. H., Shaw, G. L., Levine, L. J., Wright, E. L., Dennis, W. R., & Newcomb, R. L. (1997). Music training causes long-term enhancement of preschool children's spatial-temporal reasoning. *Neurology Research, 19*(1), 2–8.

Rauschecker, J. P. (2001). Cortical plasticity and music. *Annals of the New York Academy of Science, 930*, 330–336. Review.

Riddle, D. R., Sonntag, W. E., Lichtenwalner, R. J., 2003. Microvascular Plasticity in Aging. Aging Research Review, Apr. 2(2): 149–68.

Riddle, R. & Pollock, J. D. 2003. Making Connections: the Development of Mesencephalic Dopaninergic Neurons. Brain Research Developmental Brain Research. Dec. 30; 147(1–2): 3–21.

Ribary, U., Cappell, J., Moginer, A., Hund-Georgiadis, M., Kronberg, E., & Llinas, R. (1999). Functional images of plastic changes in the human brain. *Advances in Neurology, 81*, 49–56.

Roland, P. E. (1993). *Brain activation*. New York: Wiley-Liss, Inc.

Rosenfeld, J. P., Cha, G., Blair, T., & Gotlib, I. H. (1995). Operant (biofeedback) control of left–right frontal alpha power differences: Potential neurotherapy for affective disorders. *Biofeedback and Self-Regulation, 20*, 241–258.

Rosenzweig, M. R. (2003). Effects of differential experience on the brain and behavior. *Developmental Neuropsychology, 24*(2–3), 523–540.

Rosenzweig, M. R., & Bennett, E. L. (1996). Psychobiology of plasticity: Effects of training and experience on brain and behavior. *Behavioral Brain Research, 78*(1), 57–65.

Ross, S. T., & Soltesz, I. (2001). Long-term plasticity in interneurons of the dentate gyrus. *Proceeding of the National Academy of Sciences USA, 98*, 8874–8879.

Rowe, D. L., Robinson, P. A., & Gordon, E. (2005). Stimulant drug action in attention deficit hyperactivity disorder (ADHD): Inference of neurophysiological mechanisms via quantitative modeling. *Clinical Neurophysiology, 116*(2), 324–335.

Russell, H. L. (1996). *EEG driven audio-visual stimulation unit for enhancing cognitive abilities of learning disabled boys*. Final Report, U.S. Department of Education, Award No. 94130002.

Russell, H. L. (1997). Intellectual functioning, auditory and photic stimulation and changes in functioning in children and adults. *Biofeedback, 25*, 16–24.

Russell, H. L., & Carter, J. L. (1990). *Cognitive and behavioral changes in learning disabled children following the use of audio-visual stimulation: The Trinity Project*. Paper presented at the 16th Annual Meeting of the Biofeedback Society of Texas, Dallas, Texas.

Sakowitz, O. W., Quiroga, R. Q., Schurmann, M., & Basar, E. (2001). Bisensory stimulation increases gamma-responses over multiple cortical regions. *Brain Research, Cognitive Brain Research, 11*(2), 267–279.

Sannita, W. G. (2000). Stimulus specific oscillatory responses of the brain: A time/frequency-related coding process. *Clinical Neurophysiology, 111*, 565–583.

Sappey-Marinier, D., Calabrese, G., Fein, G., Hugg, J. W., Biggins, C., & Weiner, M. W. (1992). Effect of photic stimulation on human visual cortex lactate and phosphates using 1H and 31P magnetic resonance spectroscopy. *Journal of Cerebral Blood Flow and Metabolism, 12*, 584–592.

Schellenberg, E. G. (2004). Music lessons enhance IQ. *Psychological Science, 15*(8), 511–514.

Schellenberg, E. G. (2006). Long-Term Positive Associations Bwteen Music Lessons and IQ, *Journal of Educational Psychology*, *Vol. 98(2)*, 457–468.

Schinder, A. F., & Poo, M. (2000). The neurotrophin hypothesis for synaptic plasticity. *Trends in Neuroscience*, *23*, 639.

Schlaug, G., Norton, A., Overy, K., & Winner, E. (2005). Effects of music training on the child's brain and cognitive development. *Annals of the New York Academy of Sciences*, *1060*, 219–230.

Schmiedep, F., Louden, M., Lindenberger, U. 2010. Hundred Days of Cognitive Training Enhance Broad Cognitive Abilities: Findings from the COGITO Study. *Frontiers in Aging Neuroscience*. Pub Jul. 13:2.

Schurmann, M., & Basar, E. (2000). Oscillatory frontal theta responses are increased upon bisensory stimulations. *Clinical Neurophysiology*, *111(5)*, 884–893.

Schweitzer, J. B., Faber, T. L., Grafton, S. T., Tune, L. E., Hoffman, J. M., & Kilts, C. D. (2000). Alterations in the functional anatomy of working memory in adult attention deficit hyperactivity disorder. *Ann of J. of Psychiatry*, *157*, 278–280.

Seifert, J., Scheuerpflug, P., Zillessen, K. E., Fallgatter, A., & Warnke, A. (2003). Electro-physiological investigation of the effectiveness of methylphenidate in children with and without ADHD. *Journal of Neural Transmission*, *110(7)*, 821–829.

Shuto, S., Yoshii, K., & Matsuda, A. (2001). (1S,2R)-1-Phenyl-2-[(S)-1-aminopropyl]-N,N-diethylcyclopropanecarboxamide (PPDC), a new class of NMDA-receptor antagonist: Molecular design by a novel conformational restriction strategy. *Japanese Journal of Pharmacology*, *85(3)*, 207–213.

Sigi Hale, T., Bookheimer, S., McGough, J. J., Phillips, J. M., & McCracken, J. T. (2007). Atypical brain activation during simple and complex levels of processing in adult ADHD: An fMRI study. *Journal of Attention Disorders*, *11(2)*, 125–139. Epub May 9, 2007.

Skoe, E., & Kraus, N. (2010). Hearing it again and again: On-line subcortical plasticity in humans. *PLoS One*, *5(10)*, e13645.

Skounti, M., Philalithis, A., Mpitzaraki, K., Vamvoukas, M., & Galanakis, E. (2006). Attention-deficit/hyperactivity disorder in schoolchildren in Crete. *Acta Paediatr*, *95(6)*, 658–663.

Song, H. J., & Poo, M. (1999). Signal transduction underlying growth cone guidance by diffusible factors. *Current Opinions in Neurobiology*, *9*, 355–363.

Sonntag, W. E., Eckman, D. M., Ingralom, J. Riddle, D. R. 2007. Regulation of Cerebrovascular Aging. In Riddle, D. R., Ed., *Brain Aging: Models, Methods and Mechanisms*. Boca Raton, FL: CRC Press.

Spalletta, G., Pasini, A., Pau, F., Guido, G., Menghini, L., & Caltagirone, C. (2001). Prefrontal blood flow dysregulation in drug naive ADHD children without structural abnormalities. *Journal of Neural Transmission*, *108(10)*, 1203–1216.

Sridharan, D., Levitin, D. J., Chafe, C. H., Berger, J., & Menon, V. (2007). Neural dynamics of event segmentation in music: Converging evidence for dissociable ventral and dorsal networks. *Neuron, Aug 2;55(3)*, 521–532.

Staff, R. T., Venneri, A., Gemmell, H. G., Shanks, M. F., Pestell, S. J., & Murray, A. D. (2000). HMPAO SPECT imaging of Alzheimer's disease patients with similar content-specific autobiographic delusion: comparison using statistical parametric mapping. *Journal of Nuclear Medicine*, *41(9)*, 1451–1455.

Sterman, M. B. (1996). Physiological origins and functional correlates of EEG rhythmic activities: Implications for self-regulation. *Biofeedback and Self-Regulation*, *21*, 3–33.

Strohmenger, H. U., Lindner, K. H., Wienen, W., Vogt, J., Pulvermuller, F., Birbaumer, N., . . . Mohr, B. (1997). High frequency brain activity: Its possible role in attention perception and language processing. *Progress in Neurobiology*, *52(5)*, 427–445(19).

Sukoff, M. H. (2001). Effects of hyperbaric oxygenation. *Journal of Neurosurgery,* 95(3), 544–546.

Sun, L., Wang, Y. F., He, H., & Chen, J. (2007). Changes of the alpha competitive structure after administration of single dose methylphenidate in different subtypes of attention deficit hyperactivity disorder boys. *Beijing Da Xue Xue Bao, 39*(3), 289–292.

Suo, Z., Humphrey, J., Kundtz, A., Sethi, F., Placzek, A., Crawford, F., & Mullan, M. (1998). Soluble Alzheimer's beta-amyloid constricts the cerebral vasculature in vivo. *Neuroscience Letters, 257*(2), 77–80.

Swanson, J., Kinsbourne, M., Roberts, W., & Zucker, K. (1978). Time-response analysis of the effect of stimulant medication on the learning ability of children referred for hyperactivity. *Pediatrics, 61,* 21–29.

Swanson, J. M., Hinshaw, S. P., Arnold, L. E., Gibbons, R. D., Marcus, S., Hur, K., . . . Wigal, T. (2007). Secondary evaluations of MTA 36-month outcomes: Propensity score and growth mixture model analyses. *Journal of the American Academy of Child Adolescent Psychiatry, 46*(8), 1003–1014.

Takahashi, T., Shirane, R., Sato, S., & Yoshimoto, T. (1999). Developmental changes of cerebral blood flow and oxygen metabolism in children. *American Journal of Neuroradiology, 20*(5), 917–922.

Tansey, M. A. 1993. Ten Years Stability of EEG Biofeedback Results for a Hyperactive Boy Who Failed Fourth Grade Perceptially Impaired Class. *Biofeedback and Self Regulation.* Mar, 18(1): 33–44.

Taub, E., Griffin, A., Nick, J., Gammons, K., Uswatte, G., & Law, C. R. (2007). Pediatric CI therapy for stroke-induced hemiparesis in young children. *Developmental Neurorehabilitation, 10*(1), 3–18.

Teplan, M., Krakovska, A., & Stoic, S. (2006). EEG responses to long-term audiovisual stimulation. *International Journal of Psychophysiology, 59*(2), 81–90.

Teplan, M., Krakovska, A., & Stoic, S. (2011). Direct effects of audio-visual stimulation on EEG. *Comput Methods Programs Biomed.* Epub ahead of print.

Teplan, M., Susmakova, K., Palus, M., & Vejmelka, M. (2009). Phase synchronization in human EEG during audio-visual stimulation. *Electromagnetic Biology and Medicine 28*(1), 80–84.

Thaut, M. H. (2005). The future of music in therapy and medicine. *Annals of the New York Academy of Science, 1060,* 303–308.

Thaut, M. H. 2009. Neurologoc Music Therapy Improves Executuve Function and Emotional Adjustment in Traumatic Brain Injury Rehabilitation. *Annals of New York Academy of Sciences.* Jul. 1169: 406–16.

Thaut, M. H., Peterson, D. A., & McIntosh, G. C. (2005). Temporal entrainment of cognitive functions: Musical mnemonics induce brain plasticity and oscillatory synchrony in neural networks underlying memory. *Annals of the New York Academy of Science, 1060,* 243–254.

Thoenen, H. (1995). Neurotrophins and neuronal plasticity. *Science, 270,* 593–598.

Toga, A. W., & Thompson, P. M. (2001). Maps of the brain. *Anat Rec, 265*(2), 37–53.

Tomalski, P., & Johnson. M. H. (2010). The effects of early adversity on the adult and developing brain. *Current Opinions in Psychiatry,* March 19. Epub ahead of print.

Trainor, L. J., Shahin, A., & Roberts, L. E. (2003). Effects of musical training on the auditory cortex in children. *Annals of the New York Academy of Science, 999,* 506–513.

Visser, S. N., Lesesne, C. A., & Perou, R. (2007). National estimates and factors associated with medication treatment for childhood attention-deficit/hyperactivity disorder. *Pediatrics, 119*(Supplement 1), S99–106.

Volkow, N. D., Wang, G. J., Fowler, J. S., Logan, J., Gerasimov, M., Maynard, L., . . . Franceschi, D. (2001). Therapeutic doses of oral methylphenidate significantly increase extracellular dopamine in the human brain. *Journal of Neuroscience, 21,* RC121.

Waldron, K. A. (1995). *Introduction to a special education. The inclusive classroom.* Albany, NY: Delmar Publishers.

Wallace, M. T., & Stein, B. E. (2000). Onset of cross-modal synthesis in the neonatal superior colliculus is gated by the development of cortical influences. *Journal of Neurophysiology, 83*(6), 3578–3582.

Wallace, M. T., & Stein, B. E. (2001). Sensory and multisensory responses in the newborn monkey superior colliculus. *Journal of Neuroscience, 21*(22), 8886–8894.

Wan, C. Y., & Schlaug, G. (2010). Music making as a tool for promoting brain plasticity throughout the life span. *Neuroscientist, 16*(5), 566–577.

Wang, X., Lu, T., Snider, R. K., & Liang, L. (2005). Sustained firing in auditory cortex evoked by preferred stimuli. *Nature, 435*(7040), 341–346.

Widdig, W., Pleger, B., Rommel, O., Malin, J. P., & Tegenthoff, M. (2003). Repetitive visual stimulation: A neuropsychological approach to the treatment of cortical blindness. *NeuroRehabilitation, 18*(3), 227–237.

Wolf, S. L., Thompson, P. A., Winstein, C. J., Miller, J. P., Blanton, S. R., Nichols-Larsen, D. S., . . . Sawaki, L. (2010). The EXCITE stroke trial: comparing early and delayed constrain-induced movement therapy. *Stroke, 41*(10), 2309–2315.

Wolraich, M. L., Wibbelsman, C. J., Brown, T. E., Evans, S. W., Gotlieb, E. M., Knight J. R., . . . Wilens, T. (2005). Attention-deficit/hyperactivity disorder among adolescents: A review of the diagnosis, treatment, and clinical implications. *Pediatrics, 115*(6), 1734–1746.

Yamamoto, K., Takeuchi, Y., Tachibana, J., Uchida, K., Maeno, M., Yanashima, K., . . . Magatani, K. (2004). Analysis of brain activation by visual and auditory stimulation after visual and auditory simultaneous stimulation using fMRI. *Conference Proceedings from IEEE Engineering in Medicine and Biology Society, 3,* 1872–1875.

Yamauchi, H., Okazawa, H., Kishibe, Y., Sugimoto, K., & Takahashi, M. (2002). Changes in blood flow and oxygen metabolism during visual stimulation in carotid artery disease: Effect of baseline perfusion and oxygen metabolism. *Stroke, 33*(5), 1294–1300.

Zafra, F., Hengerer, B., Leibrock, J., Thoenen, H., & Lindholm, D. (1990). Activity dependent regulation of BDNF and NGF mRNAs in the rat hippocampus is mediated by non-NMDA glutamate receptors. *EMBO Journal, 9,* 3545–3550.

Zametkin, A. J., Nordahl, T. E., Gross, M., King, A. C., Semple, W. E., Rumsey, J., . . . Cohen, R. M. (1990). Cerebral glucose metabolism in adults with hyperactivity of childhood onset. *The New England Journal of Medicine, 323,* 1361–1366.

Zangenehpour, S., & Chaudhuri, A. (2001). Neural activity profiles of the neocortex and superior colliculus after bimodal sensory stimulation. *Cerebral Cortex, 11*(10), 924–935.

Zangenehpour, S., & Zatorre, R. J. (2010). Cross-modal of primary visual cortex following brief exposure to bimodal audiovisual stimuli. *Neuropsychologia, 48*(2), 591–600.

Zatorre, R. J. (2003). Music and the brain. *Annals of the New York Academy of Sciences, 999,* 4–14. Review.

Zatorre, R. J., Chen, J. L., & Penhune, V. B. (2007). When the brain plays music: Auditory-motor interactions in music perception and production. *National Review of Neuroscience, 8*(7), 547–558.

Ziemann, U., Muellbacher, W., Hallett, M., & Cohen, L. G. (2001). Modulation of practice-dependent plasticity in human motor cortex. *Brain, 124,* 1171–1181.

Zito, K., & Svoboda, K. (2002). Activity-dependent synaptogenesis in the adult mammalian cortex. *Neuron, 35*(6), 1015–1017. Review.

10 Conclusion

Jonathan Berger

Nearly two decades ago Judith Becker wrote (1994, p. 41): The findings of neuroscience tell us humanists something we already know. . . . But science tells us these things in a new way . . . neuroscience validates some of our most deeply held intuitions about the power of music.

Becker's pioneering and optimistic insights about the merger of science and music research lay the groundwork to explore the neurophysiological effects of music listening and music participation in the coming years. Her statement is somewhat qualified in her contribution in this volume, in which she notes that despite constant advances in the field, laboratory-based studies remain but a "diminished reflection" of the complexity of music cognition in real-world situations.

There is, perhaps, no field of research in which the inherent tension between laboratory and real-world behavioral research is more evident than research in the perception and cognition of musical rhythm. As the collective wisdom in this volume demonstrates, only by constructing a jig-saw-like puzzle, whose respective pieces comprise anthropological, musicological, and empirical scientific evidence, can one attain perspective on the phenomenon of rhythmic entrainment.

From the outset we envisioned the trajectory of this volume to be from observation and analysis of entrainment by prominent ethnomusicologists, to substantiation via imaging and physiological monitoring, to addressing potential therapeutic implications. The scholars and researchers who authored chapters in this book look at all aspects of entrainment from Becker's studies of group entrainment to Jovanov and Maxfield's study of the experience of dissociation during ritual drumming. Udo Will and Turow's detailed and thoughtful overview of entrainment, from a cognitive ethnomusicological perspective, provides a framework for Wright's generalize theory of rhythm. Whereas we avoided the temptation to incorporate tutorials in quantitative analysis, we did choose to provide a short review of principal component analysis by one of the pioneers of the method, Scott Makeig.

In addition to the inherent challenges of interdisciplinary work, the field of research on the effects of repetitive musical rhythm on the brain and nervous system risks compromise by the many entrepreneurial attempts to harness the potential therapeutic effects of rhythmic entrainment. A Google search of rhythmic entrainment returns a plethora of sites–primarily dot-coms–devoted to harnessing and commercializing complex concepts in the guise of instant healing. We thus sought a methodical, conservative, and scientific approach to considering the therapeutic implications of entrainment.

Finally, we chose to be somewhat restrictive rather than all-inclusive in our attempt to preserve a clear path through this complex and multi-faceted field. The recently invented field of 'medical ethnomusicology', for example, is not extensively represented here, but the majority of the research included in this volume intersects and informs it. We chose to maintain focus on cognitive and neurological issues, which are not typically a part of the work of these researchers, though the implications of these studies can be.

This journey began 5 years ago, when Gabe Turow, then a student in my music perception and cognition class, intrigued me with his notion of a cross-cultural view of ritual drumming and the notion that rhythmic entrainment has evolved in numerous music cultures in which trance and altered states of consciousness were integral aspects of the ritual. Over the years that followed–largely with Turow's initiative and persistence—we gathered the impressive group of scholars whose work is discussed in this volume. Seen in combination, this comprises, what we believe to be, a useful point of departure for the enormous amount of research still to be done.

REFERENCES

Becker, J. (1994). "Music and Trance." *Leonardo Music Journal, 4*, 41–51.

Contributors

ABOUT THE EDITORS

Jonathan Berger, The Denning Provostial Professor in Music, The Center for Computer Research in Music and Acoustics (CCRMA), Stanford University.

Jonathan Berger is a composer and researcher. He has composed orchestral music as well as chamber, vocal, and electro-acoustic and intermedia works. Berger was the 2010 Composer in Residence at the Spoleto USA Festival, which commissioned a chamber work for soprano Dawn Upshaw and piano quintet. Major commissions and fellowships include the National Endowment for the Arts (a work for string quartet, voice, and computer in 1984, soloist collaborations for piano, 1994, and for 'cello, 1996, and a composer's fellowship for a piano concerto in 1997); The Rockefeller Foundation (work for computer-tracked dancer, live electronics, and chamber ensemble); and The Morse and Mellon Foundations (symphonic and chamber music). Berger received prizes and commissions from the Bourges Festival, WDR, the Banff Centre for the Arts, Chamber Music America, Chamber Music Denver, the Hudson Valley Chamber Circle, The Connecticut Commission on the Arts, The Jerusalem Foundation, and others. Berger's recording of chamber music for strings, Miracles and Mud, was released by Naxos on their American Masters series in 2008. His violin concerto, Jiyeh, is available on the Gramercy Records label.

Berger's research in music perception and cognition focuses on the formulation and processing of musical expectations, and the use of music and sound to represent complex information for diagnostic and analytical purposes. He has authored and co-authored over seventy publications in music theory, computer music, sonification, audio signal processing, and music cognition.

Before joining the faculty at Stanford he taught at Yale where he was the founding director of Yale University's Center for Studies in Music

Technology. Berger was the founding Co-director of the Stan- ford Institute for Creativity and the Arts (SICA) and, co-directed the University's Arts Initiative.

Gabe Turow, Research Associate, The Center for Computer Research in Music and Acoustics and the Stanford Institute for Creativity and the Arts at Stanford University.

Following his work in the Stanford Sleep Laboratory in 2005, Turow co-designed and co-organized two symposia at Stanford on music and neuroscience. This series was annualized in 2007, supported by the Stanford Medical School, the William and Flora Hewlett Foundation, and the Stanford Institute for Creativity and the Arts. Now entering its 7th year, it is known as the Stanford Annual International Symposium Series on Music, Rhythm, and the Brain. Following his work at Stanford, with grants from Rock Against Cancer, National Music Service, and private donors, Turow helped raise $80,000 to establish the UCSF Children's Hospital Music Program. As co-director of the program, Turow provided musical instruments, bedside performances, and in-room music lessons as a means of anxiety reduction. He is currently completing work towards a music therapy license and a masters in art education at Columbia Teacher's College. Turow is also a professional instrument maker and ceramicist (StoneInstruments.com), and his work is currently on display at the Parse gallery in New Orleans. A drummer, recording artist, and music teacher, he performs regularly throughout the Bay Area.

ABOUT THE CONTRIBUTORS

Judith Becker, Professor Emeritus, School of Music, University of Michigan is the author of numerous articles and three books, *Deep Listeners: Music, Emotion, and Trancing* (2004); *Gamelan Stories: Tantrism, Islam and Aesthetics in Central Java* (1993, reprinted 2004); and *Traditional Music in Modern Java* (1980). She is the editor of *Art, Ritual and Society in Indonesia* (1979) and the three-volume set of translations entitled *Karawitan: Source Readings in Javanese Gamelan and Vocal Music* (1984, 1986, 1987). Her most recent book, *Deep Listeners: Music, Emotion, and Trancing*, received the Alan Merriam award from the Society for Ethnomusicology for the best book in ethnomusicology published during the year 2004.

Her current research focuses on the relationships between music, emotion, and ecstasy in institutionalized religious contexts and in secular contexts. She is exploring the common ground between humanistic, cultural, anthropological approaches, and scientific, cognitive, psychological approaches.

Helen K. Budzynski, Professor Emeritus, University of Washington, RN, Ph.D, is a Professor Emeritus at the University of Washington, having retired after 30 years of teaching in the Psychosocial and Community Health Department. During her years of teaching she had developed a clinic in the School of Nursing for Management of Stress Responses in which graduate student nurses were trained to perform biofeedback and to train patients to reduce or manage their chronic symptoms. Her major research was in the study of restoration of patients with cardiac and circulatory problems. Later work with her husband led to studies of neurotherapy with brain damaged and elderly patients.

Thomas Budzynski, Affiliate Professor of Psychology, University of Washington, earned a BSEE at the University of Detroit and served as an aerospace inertial systems engineer on the SR-71 Blackbird project at Area 51. He later went back to academia to gain a masters and Ph.D. in psychology. As a grad student in the mid '60s, Dr. Budzynski invented one of the first EMG biofeedback systems. In 1970, Dr. Budzynski developed the Twilight Learner, one of the first neurotherapy systems. He was elected President of the Biofeedback Research Society in 1974. In the last few years he has returned to teaching and neurotechnology research at the University of Washington in Seattle. There, with his wife Helen Budzynski, he is conducts studies on AVS (audio-visual stimulation) effects on the brain, priming effects of binaural tones on the EEG, chronic fatigue syndrome, applications to chronic pain, enhanced academic performance, and the enhancement of cognitive process in head-injured, learning-disordered, and elderly patients.

He has lectured and headed workshops on these topics in many foreign countries as well as the U.S. In 1999 he received the Distinguished Scientist Award from the Association for Applied Psychophysiology and Biofeedback at their annual meeting in Vancouver, B.C., Canada. In 2002, he received a Career Achievement award from the International Society for Neuronal Research. At present, he is an Affiliate Professor at the University of Washington and co-editing *Introduction to Quantitative EEG and Neurofeedback, Advanced Theory and Applications, 2nd Edition* for Elsevier. He is a licensed psychologist in the State of Washington and maintains an active private practice of neurotherapy and biofeedback in his clinic in Poulsbo, WA, where he uses neurofeedback therapy (Z-Score Training) with clients suffering from learning disorders, traumatic head injury, depression, and anxiety.

Emil Jovanov, Associate Professor, Electrical and Computer Engineering, University of Alabama in Huntsville. His research interests include wearable physiological monitoring, ubiquitous and mobile computing, biomedical signal processing, and physiological modeling. He serves as Associate Editor of the IEEE Transactions on Information Technology in Biomedicine, IEEE Transactions on Biomedical Circuits and Systems, and International Journal of Telemedicine and Applications (IJTA), Editorial Board member of Applied Psychophysiology and Biofeedback, and served as a Program Secretary of the International Symposium and Workshop on Scientific Bases of Consciousness in 1997.

Dr. Jovanov has been working on physiological correlates and models of altered states of consciousness for more than 10 years. He investigated autonomous nervous system and brain activity during meditation, relaxation techniques, musicogenic states, and healer/healee interactions. Dr. Jovanov developed several environments for processing, visualization, and perceptualization of physiological signals.

James D. Lane, Associate Research Professor of Medical Psychology and Behavioral Medicine; Director, DUMC Psychophysiology Laboratory, Duke University. He is professor of medical psychology in the Department of Psychiatry and Behavioral Sciences at Duke University Medical Center, where he directs the Psychophysiology Laboratory. He has worked for more than 30 years in the fields of psychophysiology and behavioral medicine, exploring the harmful effects of stress and developing new ideas that individuals can use to reduce stress and improve health. His interest in rhythmic stimulation and binaural beats emerges from his interest in technologies that people can use to improve their lives.

Scott Makeig, Director, Swartz Center for Computational Neuroscience, Institute for Neural Computation, University of California, San Diego. He received a Ph.D. in Music Psychobiology from the University of California San Diego (UCSD) in 1985. After spending a year in Ahmednagar, India, as an American India Foundation research fellow, he became a research psychobiologist at UCSD, and then a research psychologist at the Naval Health Research Center, San Diego. In 1999, he joined the Salk Institute, La Jolla, as a senior staff scientist, and moved to UCSD as a Research Scientist in 2002 to develop the Swartz Center for Computational Neuroscience, which he now directs, under the UCSD Institute for Neural Computation. His research interests are in developing and applying new methods for observing and modeling distributed human brain dynamics supporting active agency, including artistic expression, and creativity. An amateur musician, he plays piano, folk guitar, and is currently attempting to play traditional Irish music on the violin. He also composes and arranges songs and, most recently, a 10-minute suite for the Swartz

Center's own Sino-Celtic Orchestra, for performance at the UCSD Chancellor's reception for the Swartz Center benefactor in 2006.

Melinda C. Maxfield, Researcher, Institute of Transpersonal Psychology, Palo Alto, CA; Vice President of the Maxfield Foundation. He specializes in cross-cultural health care methodologies and research on the physical and psychological effects of percussion. Melinda's research includes a pilot study at the Lucille Packard Children's Hospital at Stanford, Oncology Unit, in collaboration with Dr. Frank Lawless and Dr. Jeanne Achterberg, on non-medicated pain management and immune system enhancement. She has traveled to Tuva (S. Siberia, Russia), as a representative of the Foundation for Shamanic Studies, where she presented a paper at the International Conference on Shamanism and engaged in field research with Tuvinian shamans. She is currently involved in various projects that apply traditional shamanic techniques, such as the shamanic journey and rhythmic drumming, to work with depression, chronic pain, and issues related to terminal illness. In Buenos Aires, at the Fundacion Argentino-Brasileira (a center to aid those in life-crisis), and in Germany, she conducts seminars to facilitate physical, mental, and emotional well-being and to enhance the quality of life. Melinda has worked with Angeles Arrien for 7 years, and now assists her at the Four Fold Way residential trainings. She is Vice President of the Maxfield Foundation, an organization to support cancer research, and is on the board of the Foundation for Shamanic Studies, the Angeles Arrien Foundation for Cross-Cultural Education and Research, and the Amazon Conservation Team (ACT).

Leslie H. Sherlin, On faculty at the University of Phoenix, the Southwest College of Naturopathic Medicine, and Northern Arizona University. She is on faculty at the University of Phoenix, the Southwest College of Naturopathic Medicine, and Northern Arizona University. He is the director of QEEG Rapid Reporting Services at Q-Metrx, Inc., the President of Nova Tech EEG, Inc., and a Quantitative Electroencephalograph Diplomate. He is an expert in the analysis of the LORETA EEG mapping technique, having served as a laboratory research assistant to Dr. Joel Lubar at the University of Tennessee.

Hsin Yi Tang, Assistant Professor at College of Nursing, Seattle University, Ph.D., APRN-BC., is an Assistant Professor at College of Nursing, Seattle University. She is a psychiatric mental health nurse practitioner. Her research focus is on mind–body health promotion/rehabilitation through alternative approaches, such as neurofeedback training for head injury, light–sound stimulation for cognitive enhancement, and music therapy for stress management and cardiac health. Her other expertise is instrument/questionnaire design and development. Dr. Tang's current research grant is funded by John L. Locke Jr. Charitable Trust in Perpetuity; it was awarded for a randomized controlled study aiming to evaluate the short-term and long-term effect of two audio relaxation programs on blood pressure reduction in older adults.

Concetta M. Tomaino, Executive Director, Institute for Music and Neurologic Function, and Senior Vice President, Music Therapy Services, Beth Abraham Family of Health Service, D.A., MT-BC, LCAT, is the executive director and co-founder of the Institute for Music and neurologic function and senior vice president for music therapy at Beth Abraham Family of Health Services, Bronx, NY. Dr. Tomaino has had a 28-year career at Beth Abraham, including helping to create the Institute for Music and Neurologic Function, a center to restore, maintain, and improve peoples' physical, emotional, and neurologic functioning through the systematic use of music. Dr. Tomaino's clinical practice is specialized in the use of music therapy for individuals with Alzheimer's disease, Parkinson's disease and other neurological diseases. Internationally known for her research in the clinical applications of music, she lectures on music therapy throughout the world and has authored numerous articles. Currently, Dr. Tomaino teaches at the Albert Einstein College of Medicine and the Brookdale Center of Aging at Hunter College.

Harold Russell, Former Adjunct Research Professor, Department of Gerontology and Health Promotion, The University of Texas Medical Branch at Galveston, earned his M.S. and Ph.D. in Clinical Psychology at the University of Houston. During a 2-year clinical residency at the University of Texas Medical Branch—Galveston, he began to explore ways of reducing the high levels of stress and anxiety that interfered with the school performance of children and of medical students. For 15 years he continued this research while remaining on the faculty in the Department of Psychiatry and Behavioral Sciences.

He conducted pioneering work using biofeedback and neurofeedback during the 1970s as tools to teach both children and adults to control their anxieties and improve their school performance. When administrative changes occurred, Dr. Russell began an 18-year private practice in Galveston focused on both stress disorders and learning problems. Since ending his practice, he has devoted most of his time and energies to exploring ways to increase children's abilities to learn using therapeutic tools that are inexpensive enough to be available to nearly everyone.

Udo Will, Professor of Ethnomusicology at Ohio State University, studied music, sociology, and neuroscience. He holds Ph.D.s in both musicology and neurobiology and is professor of cognitive ethnomusicology at Ohio State University. He currently leads research projects on cognitive aspects of music performances in oral cultures, on rhythm and melody processing by the human brain, and on a comparison of the cognitive architecture of music and language production. He is co-founder, together with Martin Clayton (Milton Keynes) and Ian Cross (Cambridge), of the Music and Entrainment Network, an international research group sponsored by a 3-year grant from the British Academy.

Dr. Matthew Wright is a media systems designer, improvising composer/musician and computer music researcher. He plays a variety of traditional plucked lutes, Afro- Brazilian percussion, and computer-based instruments of his own design, in both traditional music contexts and experimental new works. He was the Musical Systems Designer at U.C. Berkeley's Center for New Music and Audio Technology (CNMAT) from 1993–2008, and is known for his promotion of the Sound Description Interchange Format (SDIF) and Open Sound Control (OSC) standards, as well as his work with real- time mapping of musical gestures to sound synthesis. His dissertation at Stanford's Center for Computer Research in Music and Acoustics (CCRMA) concerned computer modeling of the perception of musical rhythm: "The Shape of an Instant: Measuring and Modeling Perceptual Attack Time with Probability Density Functions." After one year as a visiting research fellow at the University of Victoria on the theme of "Computational Ethnomusicology" he is now the Research Director at UC Santa Barbara's Center for Research in Electronic Arts and Technology (CREATE) and the Principal Development Engineer for the AlloSphere, a 3-story full-surround immersive audiovisual instrument for scientific and artistic research.

Index